THE HORSE IN MOTION

Sarah Pilliner

Samantha Elmhurst

Zoe Davies

Blackwell
Science

© 2002 by Blackwell Science Ltd, a Blackwell
Publishing Company
Editorial Offices:
Osney Mead, Oxford OX2 0EL, UK
  Tel: +44 (0)1865 206206
Blackwell Science, Inc., 350 Main Street,
Malden, MA 02148-5018, USA
  Tel: +1 781 388 8250
Iowa State Press, a Blackwell Publishing
Company, 2121 State Avenue, Ames, Iowa
50014-8300, USA
  Tel: +1 515 292 0140
Blackwell Publishing Asia Pty Ltd, 550
Swanston Street, Carlton South, Melbourne,
Victoria 3053, Australia
  Tel: +61 (0)3 9347 0300
Blackwell Wissenschafts Verlag,
Kurfürstendamm 57, 10707 Berlin, Germany
  Tel: +49 (0)30 32 79 060

First published 2002 by Blackwell Science Ltd

Library of Congress
Cataloging-in-Publication Data
Pilliner, Sarah
    The horse in motion/Sarah Pilliner,
    Samantha Elmhurst, Zoe Davies
    p. cm.
    ISBN 0-632-05137-X
    Horses – paces, gaits, etc.   2. Horses –
    anatomy.   I. Elmhurst, Samantha.
    II. Davies, Zoe.   III. Title.

    SF289 .P56 2002
    636.1'089276-dc21
                                    2001052688

ISBN 0-632-05137-X

A catalogue record for this title is available
from the British Library

Set in 10/13 pt Palatino
by SNP Best-set Typesetter Ltd., Hong Kong
Printed and bound in Great Britain by
The Alden Press, Oxford
and Northampton

For further information on
Blackwell Science, visit our website:
www.blackwell-science.com

Contents

Preface

We all want our horses to be able to perform to the best of their ability and we know that an effective training regime has many facets. The horse must be worked correctly, fed a balanced ration, mentally and physically healthy and well looked after. This book examines a further aspect of the horse's performance: it is designed to help all horse owners and riders to understand how a horse moves and how its anatomy helps, or hinders, the horse's athletic ability.

No horse has perfect conformation, but no matter what their physical characteristics all horses have the same biomechanical function. The better the horse's conformation and physique the more efficient it will be in biomechanical terms. In simple terms the horse will find it easier to do the job and, as a result, will put less stress and strain on the muscles, bones, tendons, ligaments and joints so will be likely to stay sounder for longer. As the demands of competition increase, it is inevitable that success will depend upon attention to the finest detail; for example, individualised work and exercise programmes, development of the horses' physical capacity for work, prevention and treatment of injury and speedy and effective recovery from exertion. Having more knowledge about how their horse moves and the things that it finds easy or difficult to do allows the rider to develop a work regime involving specific exercises that will enhance the horse's performance and prolong its working life. It will also help riders recognise the limitations imposed on performance by the horse's own physical make-up.

This book examines horse anatomy, and then considers the phases of the horse's gaits, using sequences of photographs and detailed anatomical drawings to show the systems of support and movement at each phase. The walk, trot, canter, gallop and jump are all examined, and the effect of the rider on the horse evaluated so that the rider can take appropriate action to avoid hindering the horse. Tips are provided throughout on ways in which the horse's life can be made easier, such as saddle fitting, warming up and cooling down procedures.

Ultimately, it is up to the rider to be sensitive to the individual requirements of his or her horse and to devise a programme of exercise and training that best suits the individual animal, taking into account its conformation, movement and action and its mental and physical ability to cope with the work.

Part 1

Anatomy and Conformation

Chapter 1

The whole horse

Introduction (Fig. 1.1)

This book is designed to help all horse owners and riders understand how a horse moves and how its anatomy helps it to perform. It will also help riders recognise the limitations imposed on performance by the horse's own physical make-up.

Contrary to popular belief the horse, although a natural athlete, is not a natural jumper. A loose horse, given enough excitement, will naturally perform movements that equate to passage, piaffe, courbette and capriole; however, the horse's heavy gut and relatively inflexible spine combine to make jumping more difficult. Figure 1.1 shows the template of the whole horse used for illustrative purposes throughout this book.

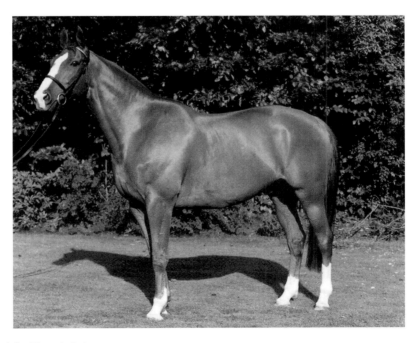

Fig. 1.1 The whole horse

Training the performance horse

Observation of the following points when exercising and training the performance horse will help to protect bones, tendons, ligaments and muscles from injury:

- Feeding a balanced diet will ensure that the necessary nutrients for energy production, and tissue maintenance and repair are available.
- Water is essential to maintain all body functions; therefore a supply of fresh clean water must be available.
- The salts lost in sweat should be replaced in the form of electrolytes in the diet; these body salts are vital for nerve and muscle function.
- Thorough warming up before executing strenuous or difficult exercises will ensure adequate blood supply to the muscles and minimise the rise of injury.
- Thorough cooling down after exercise will help the circulation remove the toxic waste products of exercise (for example, lactic acid) and reduce muscle stiffness.
- Allowing the horse periods of relaxation and stretching during work will help to prevent tension. When muscles are held in tension (think how your shoulders feel after a stressful drive) the blood supply is inadequate to remove waste products which accumulate and increase the risk of injury and stiffness.
- Regular shoeing to keep the horse's feet in balance will ensure that the joints of the limb remain in correct alignment and that the forces generated during work are transmitted up the limb in a way that minmises the risk of injury.

Points of the horse (Fig. 1.2)

Familiarity with the surface anatomy of the horse is important so that underlying structures can be identified. The horse has evolved over many thousands of years from a small fox-like creature with four toes on each foot to the animal it is today with a single hoof at the end of each limb. Figure 1.2 shows the points of the horse in detail.

The skeleton (Fig. 1.3)

The skeleton is the framework that supports and protects the soft tissues of the horse's body. In Fig. 1.2 many bony areas lying below the skin are identified. Figure 1.3 shows the positions of the bones that give rise to some of the points of the horse.

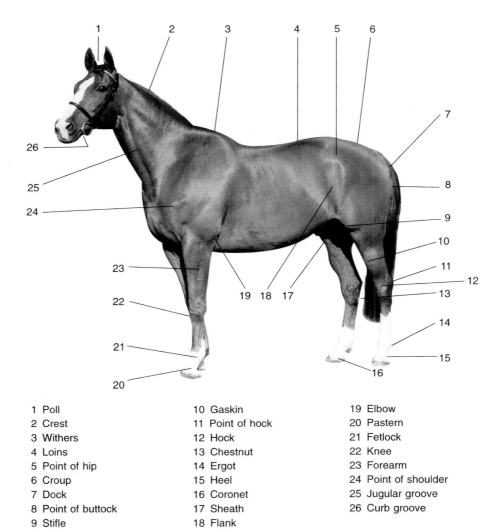

Fig. 1.2 Points of the horse

1 Poll	10 Gaskin	19 Elbow
2 Crest	11 Point of hock	20 Pastern
3 Withers	12 Hock	21 Fetlock
4 Loins	13 Chestnut	22 Knee
5 Point of hip	14 Ergot	23 Forearm
6 Croup	15 Heel	24 Point of shoulder
7 Dock	16 Coronet	25 Jugular groove
8 Point of buttock	17 Sheath	26 Curb groove
9 Stifle	18 Flank	

Functions of the skeleton

- The skeleton is made of bone.
- Bone protects soft tissue; for example, the skull encloses and protects the brain, and the vertebral column encloses and protects the spinal cord.
- Skeletal muscles are attached to bones via tendons to enable movement.
- Bone is a living tissue with a supply of blood and nerves.
- Bones meet and articulate at joints that vary in their ability to move.

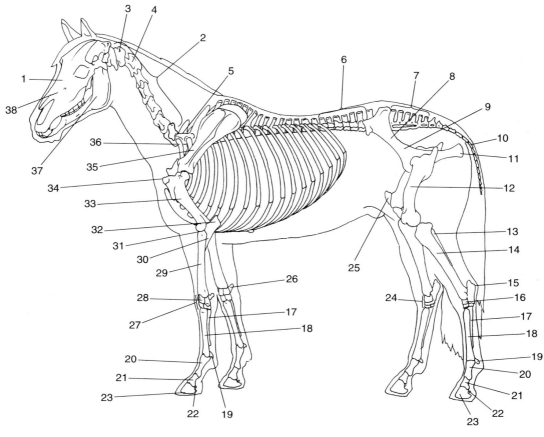

Fig. 1.3 Skeleton

1 Skull
2 Seven cervical vertebrae
3 Atlas
4 Axis
5 First thoracic vertebra
6 Lumbar vertebrae
7 Sacral vertebrae
8 Ilium
9 Pelvis
10 Coccygeal vertebrae
11 Point of buttock (ischium)
12 Femur
13 Fibula
14 Tibia
15 Point of hock
16 Hock
17 Splint bone
18 Cannon bone
19 Proximal sesamoid bones

20 Long pastern
21 Short pastern
22 Navicular bone
23 Pedal bone
24 Tarsal bones
25 Patella
26 Pisiform bone
27 Carpal bones
28 Knee
29 Radius
30 Ulna
31 Elbow
32 Olecranon process
33 Humerus
34 Point of shoulder
35 Scapula
36 First rib
37 Mandible
38 Maxilla

- The ends of the bones making up movable joints are covered by cartilage, allowing them to slide smoothly over one another.
- Ligaments bind bone to bone, supporting the joints.
- The interior of the joint is lubricated by synovial fluid which is secreted by the membrane covering the cartilage at the ends of the bones.

Skeletal muscles

The horse's skeleton is incapable of movement on its own. All movements, from a flick of the tail to the most difficult dressage manoeuvre, are brought about by a complicated system of skeletal muscles. All horses, regardless of breed, size or age, have the same arrangement of skeletal muscles, but some muscles may be better developed in certain horses depending upon their type of training. For example, the Thoroughbred dressage horse will have a more highly developed topline than a racing-fit Thoroughbred. In addition, centuries of selective breeding have led to enhanced muscular development in some breeds and types of horses. The Quarter horse, bred to sprint over a quarter of a mile, has highly muscular forelimbs and hindquarters. The sprinting Thoroughbred naturally has a more muscular physique than its steeplechasing counterpart.

The skeletal muscles are under the horse's conscious control and enable it to adjust to the surrounding environment and to make necessary movements such as running or grazing. Muscles are attached to and hence move, various parts of the skeleton and body.

Skeletal muscles create movement by acting across joints. They are usually arranged in opposing groups which perform opposite actions to give smooth and even movements. *Flexors* are placed behind the bone and pull it backwards, i.e. bend the joint, whereas *extensors* are placed in front of the bone and pull it forwards, i.e. straighten the joint from the bent position. Usually one of the pair of muscles is much stronger than the other.

Each end of the muscle tapers from a larger muscle belly into a tendon, which attaches the muscle to the bone. Muscle bellies vary in size and shape: some are large flat sheets, such as the latissimus dorsi, and others are long and strap-like, such as the brachiocephalicus.

The horse has no muscles below the knee, and all movement in this area is carried out via tendons attached to the muscles higher up the limb. This results in the lower limbs of performance horses being prone to tendon and ligament injury. Tired muscles are more likely to result in injury.

For muscles to produce movement, they must be attached to bone at both ends. These ends are sometimes classified as the 'origin' and 'insertion', the origin being the less movable of the two ends. In most cases, when the muscle contracts (shortens) the insertion end is brought closer to the origin.

Muscles use energy to contract but do not have a way of stretching themselves again: instead the contraction of the opposing muscle is used to lengthen the shortened muscle. For example, if the splenius at the top of the neck contracts, the head is lifted and the sternocephalicus on the underside of the neck is lengthened correspondingly.

There are approximately 700 separate skeletal muscles in the horse's body. The name of the muscle may tell us what the main action of that muscle is; for example, the digital extensor extends the toe. Others, however, are named after their places of attachment; for example, the brachiocephalicus extends from the arm (brachium) to the head (cephalicus). Names of some muscles and their actions are listed in Table 1.1.

The muscles can be considered as belonging to two systems:

- The superficial muscles which lie just below the skin
- The deep muscles which lie underneath the superficial muscles.

The superficial muscles are shown in Fig. 1.4 and the deep musculature is shown in Fig. 1.5.

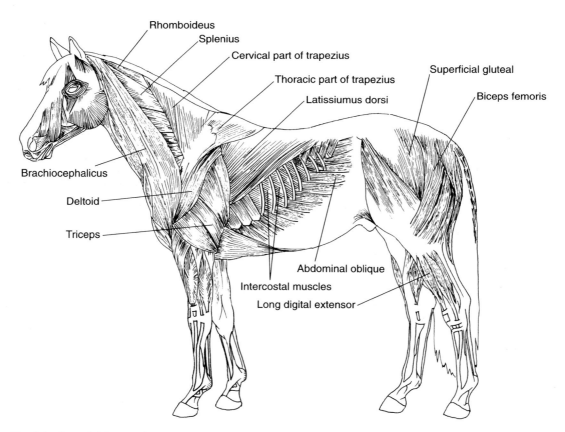

Fig. 1.4 Superficial musculature

Table 1.1 Muscle actions

Muscle name	Origin	Insertion	Action
Trapezius (thoracis)	Thoracic vertebrae	Scapula	Lifts shoulder
Trapezius (cervicis)	Cervical vertebrae	Scapula	Lifts shoulder
Splenius	Spines of 4th and 6th thoracic vertebrae	Wing of atlas and cervical vertebrae	Elevates head and turns head and neck to one side
Sternocephalicus	Sternum	Back of jaw	Flexes head and neck forwards and downwards
Rhomboideus	Occiput	Top of scapula	Lifts shoulder upwards and forwards
Brachiocephalicus	Wing of atlas	Humerus	Acts on cervical vertebrae, extends the shoulder and produces sideways movement of head and neck
Supraspinatus	Scapula	Humerus	Advances the forelimb
Deep pectoral	Sternum	Humerus	Helps raise thorax relative to the limb
Deltoideus	Scapula	Humerus	Flexes shoulder joint
Latissimus dorsi	Thoracic spines, withers	Humerus	Flexes the shoulder joint and retracts forelimb
Serratus ventralis	Ribs (lateral surfaces of 1st to 9th)	Scapula	Lifts body in relation to the scapula; suspends trunk between scapulae
Biceps femoris	Sacral vertebrae	Femur (3rd trochanter)	Extends and abducts the hind limb; propulsion, rearing and kicking
Semitendinosus (make up the hamstring group)	Pelvis (tuber ischii and ilium)	Tibia	Extends hip and hock and flexes the stifle so that limb is rotated inwards and provides propulsion
Semimembranosus	Pelvis	Femur stifle (medial side)	Adducts hind limb
Gluteus	Pelvis	Femur (trochanter major)	Abducts limb, strong hip extensor; rearing, kicking and propulsion
Longissimus dorsi	Pelvis (sacrum)	Thoracic vertebrae	Transmits propulsion from the hind limbs
Digital extensors	Upper ends of radius and ulna	Via tendons to long pastern, short pastern and pedal bone	Carries limb and foot forwards
Digital flexors	Upper ends of radius and ulna	Via tendons to short pastern and pedal bone	Flexes the knee, fetlock and foot

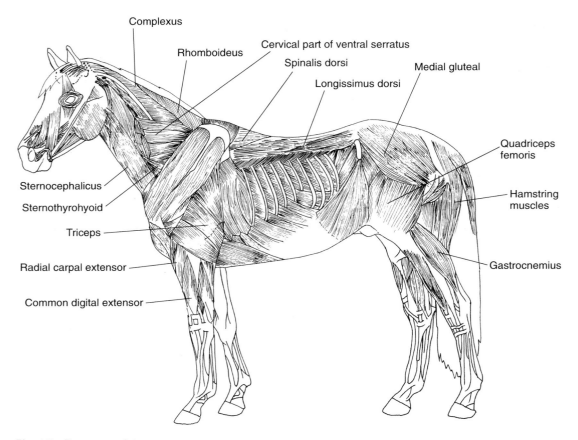

Fig. 1.5   Deep musculature

Chapter 2

The head and neck

Introduction

The horse's head acts as a heavy weight that is suspended at the end of a long neck (Fig. 2.1). This arrangement allows the horse to alter its centre of gravity with ease. The position of the horse's head and neck has a significant effect on balance and weight distribution; this is discussed in more detail in Chapter 8. When the horse's head and neck are lowered, more weight is carried on the forelimbs and the centre of gravity moves forward. When the head and neck are raised, more weight is carried on the hind limbs and the centre of gravity moves back. Muscles originating in the forelimb and trunk that have a critical role in forelimb movement are attached to the neck bones.

The skull (Fig. 2.2)

The skull is made up of many flat bones fitted together like a jigsaw puzzle. These are connected together by fibrous joints known as sutures, which ossify (become bone) with age. The junctions between the bones of the skull become indistinct with age. The function of the skull is to protect very delicate organs such as the brain and eyes, and other vital sensory organs such as the nose and ears.

The eyes are situated deep within the orbits, offering them some degree of protection. They each sit in a pad of fat which provides a cushioning effect. When horses are ill or starving this fat disappears and the eyes appear more sunken.

The skin which covers the horse's face and neck is thinner than the skin anywhere else on the body.

Teeth

The horse's head evolved to be relatively large in relation to the overall size of the animal. This was due to changes in dietary habits, which developed with time from shrub browsing to a trickle-feeding

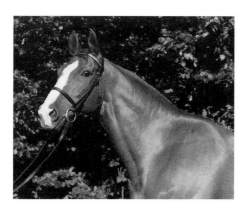

Fig. 2.1 The head and neck

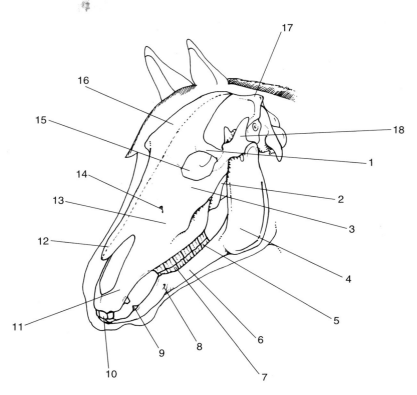

1 Zygomatic process of the frontal bone
2 Temporal bone
3 Facial crest
4 Mandible
5 Premolars
6 Ramus of mandible
7 Molars
8 Mental foramen
9 Canine tooth (tush)
10 Incisor teeth
11 Incisive bone (premaxilla)
12 Nasal bone
13 Maxilla
14 Infraorbital foramen
15 Orbit
16 Cranium
17 Nuchal crest
18 Zygomatic arch

Fig. 2.2 Skeleton of the head and neck

herbivore. The horse needed large teeth for grinding herbage and consequently a large jawbone to accommodate them. All the lower teeth are situated in the mandible. The upper teeth are situated in sockets in the incisive (premaxillary) and maxillary bones.

The horse's teeth are designed to cope with a diet mainly consisting of grass, grinding away at tough stems and leaves. To compensate for the continual wear that occurs at their grinding (occlusal) surfaces, the horse's teeth possess a very long crown, most of which is embedded in a socket. As the tooth is worn away the crown gradually emerges from the socket, compensating for the wear. The horse's jaws need to be long to house this battery of grinding teeth; they also need to be deep to encase the long, embedded crowns. This gives rise to the characteristic shape of the horse's head.

Tooth care

To assist the grinding process, the upper jaw is wider than the bottom jaw and the surfaces of the teeth comprise complex folds of enamel. The side-to-side chewing action of the jaws means that the teeth glide across each other, with continual eruption compensating for wear. Through generations of selective breeding, horse's heads have become more refined, with the Thoroughbred and Arab clearly possessing a wide forehead and top jaw and a narrower lower jaw. When the upper jaw is wider than the bottom jaw, the chewing action does not involve the entire occlusal surface of the tooth. The inside of the upper molars is worn smooth while the outside is not sufficiently worn away, leaving sharp edges that can damage the horse's cheeks. The outside edge of the lower teeth is worn but the inside edges become sharp and can lacerate the tongue. The situation is made even worse when horses are fed lower levels of fibrous roughage and larger amounts of easily chewed concentrate feed. The horse's teeth should be checked twice a year by a horse dentist or veterinary surgeon, and if necessary rasped to remove these sharp edges.

The neck

The skeleton of the horse's neck consists of seven cervical vertebrae (Fig. 2.3), the first of which is the atlas (Fig. 2.4) and the second the axis (Fig. 2.5). The long strong ligament of the neck, the nuchal ligament (Fig. 2.7), is attached to the axis. It helps to support the horse's heavy head and neck, and allows them to be raised and lowered. The joints between the other cervical vertebrae enable the horse to stretch the neck downwards, bend it sideways and arch it. This allows the horse to graze and to move its head towards strange sounds or sights which may indicate danger. The curves formed by the vertebrae are deep in the neck and do not follow the crest.

Cervical vertebrae

The first two bones of the horse's neck, the atlas and axis, are different anatomically from the other neck vertebrae and also from each other. The hollow space within these vertebrae, which allows the vital spinal cord to run through their middle, is relatively large to allow for the great amount of movement which takes place in this part of the neck.

Atlas (Fig. 2.4)

The atlas consists of a short tube of bone with large wings; it lacks the body of the axis and other cervical vertebrae. It articulates with the skull at the occiput, allowing the horse to nod its head. The wings of the atlas

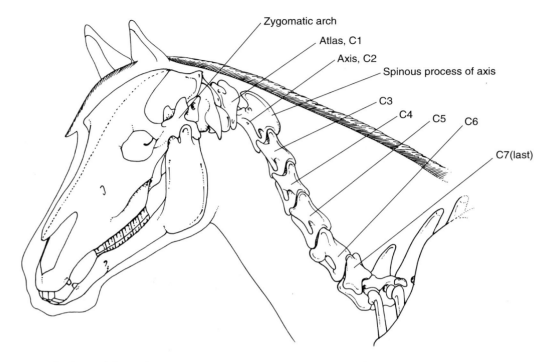

Fig. 2.3 Skeleton of the neck

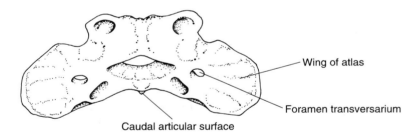

Fig. 2.4 Atlas – dorsal view

can be felt on either side of the horse's neck below the poll and behind the jawbone.

Axis (Fig. 2.5)

The axis is attached to the atlas by a tooth-like projection, known as the odontoid process, which allows the head to move from side to side. The upper surface of the odontoid process is uneven to allow the attachment of a strong ligament which maintains its joint to the atlas. The atlas also has a large dorsal spinous process to allow attachment of neck muscles and the important nuchal ligament, the strong central ligament of the neck.

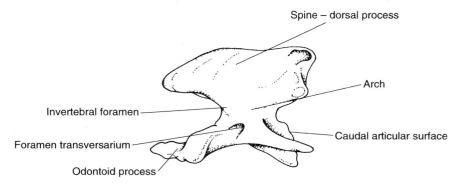

Spine – dorsal process

Arch

Invertebral foramen

Caudal articular surface

Foramen transversarium

Odontoid process

Fig. 2.5   Axis – lateral view

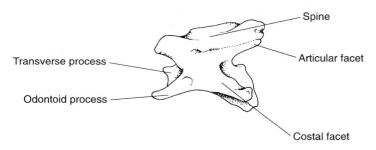

Spine

Articular facet

Transverse process

Odontoid process

Costal facet

Fig. 2.6   Cervical vertebra – lateral view

Cervical vertebrae C3–C7 (Fig. 2.6)

Cervical vertebrae C3–C7 have much reduced spinous processes. They have transverse processes which project sideways; again, these enable muscular attachment, for example of the serratus ventralis muscle (see Fig. 2.8). The ligaments associated with the vertebrae include the supraspinous ligament, which runs along the top of the spinous processes of the vertebrae and unites the summits of all lumbar and thoracic vertebrae.

Nuchal ligament (Fig. 2.7)

The nuchal ligament (ligamentum nuchae) supports and holds the horse's head and neck in position. It consists of two parts:

• The funicular part is a rope-like ligament which supports the head and runs along the top of the neck.
• The lamellar part is a band attaching to the cervical vertebrae, which restrains the movement of the dorsal spines and supports the weight of the head.

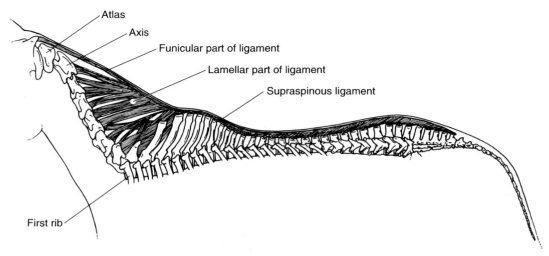

Fig. 2.7 Nuchal ligament

The funicular part is a continuation of the supraspinous ligament which runs along the back from the sacrum. It attaches to the dorsal spines of all the lumbar and thoracic vertebrae and helps to keep these bones in line.

Superficial and deep musculature (Figs 2.8, 2.9)

Facial muscles

There are many facial muscles directly associated with the horse's eyes, ears, nostrils and mouth. These muscles originate on the bones of the face and cranium; they produce expression of the face and allow the horse to prick the ears, flare the nostrils or bare the teeth. The eyes are supplied with three lids, the normal upper and lower lids plus a third eyelid. The masseter forms the basis of the cheek and is responsible for closing the jaw.

Brachiocephalicus

The brachiocephalicus is a long flattened muscle arising from the mastoid process of the temporal bone behind the ear. This muscle runs down the length of the neck, inserting onto the humerus; it forms the upper boundary of the jugular groove. The brachiocephalicus muscle acts on the cervical vertebrae, extends the shoulder and produces sideways movement of the head and neck.

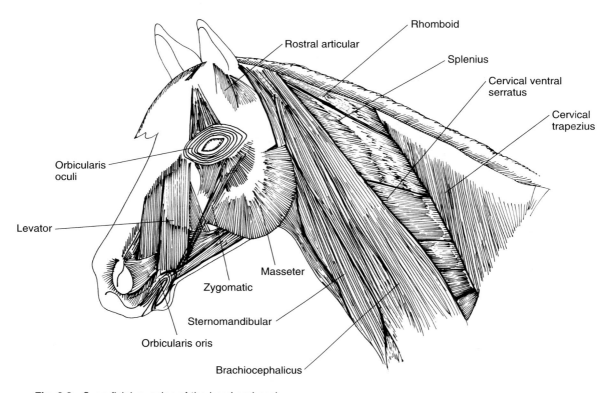

Fig. 2.8   Superficial muscles of the head and neck

Trapezius

The cervical part of the trapezius runs from the cervical vertebrae to the scapula and is a flattened, triangular sheet of superficial muscle. It draws the scapula up and back to lift the shoulder.

Splenius

The splenius originates at the thoracic vertebrae and inserts into the wing of the atlas and cervical vertebrae. This muscle flexes the cervical vertebrae to lift and turn the head from side to side.

Sternocephalicus

The sternocephalicus is long and narrow, and runs from the sternum to the jaw; it forms the boundary of the jugular groove. This muscle flexes the horse's head and neck forward and down.

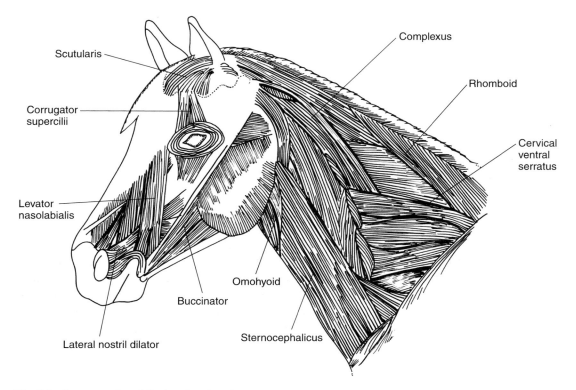

Scutularis

Corrugator
supercilii

Levator
nasolabialis

Lateral nostril dilator

Buccinator

Omohyoid

Sternocephalicus

Complexus

Rhomboid

Cervical
ventral
serratus

Fig. 2.9   Deep muscles of the head and neck

Rhomboideus

Underneath the trapezius muscle lies the cervical part of the rhomboideus. This muscle originates in the occiput and inserts into the top of the scapula. The rhomboideus lifts the shoulder up and forward.

Chapter 3

The forelimb

Introduction

As the horse evolved into a fleet-footed herbivore, the proportions of the limbs changed. To achieve greater speed the lower limb was kept as light as possible; thus the horse has no muscle below the knee or the hock. The pull of the muscles higher up the leg is transmitted to the bones of the lower leg and foot by long tendons which can easily be felt by running one's fingers down the back of the horse's leg. The length and position of these tendons means that they are susceptible to damage and injury. The design of the forelimb ensures that forces are conducted in a straight line up and down the limb, so that one structure is not stressed more than another.

Design and function (Fig. 3.1)

In reality the modern horse stands on the tip of the middle digit of each forelimb and the tip of the middle toe of each hind limb. The hoof, which is similar to a human nail, has developed to protect the end of each limb; it also acts as a shock absorber. The horse's forelimb is attached to the body by muscles and ligaments; there is no bony attachment or collarbone equivalent. This influences both the horse's movement and the way in which the forelimbs absorb concussion. In the standing horse, 60% of the weight of the body is carried by the forelimbs and they have to withstand the majority of the impact experienced during movement. Forelimbs are designed not only to act as shock absorbers; they also have an important role in moving off and propulsion which will be discussed later.

The skeleton (Figs 3.2–3.4)

The forelimb consists of the following bones:

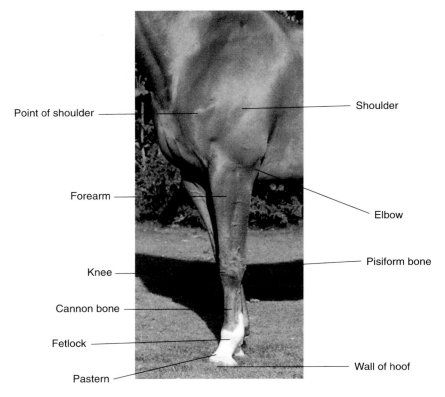

Point of shoulder ——
Shoulder ——
Forearm ——
Elbow ——
Knee ——
Pisiform bone ——
Cannon bone ——
Fetlock ——
Wall of hoof ——
Pastern ——

Fig. 3.1 Side view of the forelimb

- Scapula
- Humerus
- Radius
- Ulna
- Knee or carpus (consisting of seven or eight carpal bones)
- Cannon (large metacarpal) bone
- Two splint bones (medial and small metacarpals)
- Long pastern (first phalanx)
- Short pastern (second phalanx)
- Pedal bone (third phalanx)
- Two proximal sesamoid bones
- Navicular bone (distal sesamoid bone).

Scapula

The scapula is a triangular flattened bone which glides over the rib cage. The length and angulation of the scapula (ideally 45°) determine the slope of the horse's shoulder and the length of stride. The thorax is slung between the two scapulae by an arrangement of muscles, tendons and ligaments known as the thoracic sling.

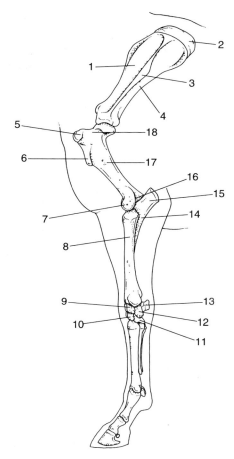

Fig. 3.2   Skeleton of the forelimb – side view

1 Supraspinous fossa
2 Scapular cartilage
3 Spine of the scapula
4 Infraspinous fossa
5 Greater tubercule (lateral tuberosity)
6 Deltoid tuberosity
7 Lateral condyle
8 Radius
9 Intermediate carpal bone

10 Third carpal bone
11 Fourth carpal bone
12 Ulnar carpal bone
13 Accessory carpal bone (pisiform)
14 Ulna
15 Olecranon tuber
16 Olecranon fossa
17 Humerus
18 Humeral head

Humerus

The shoulder is a ball and socket joint (the type of joint that allows the greatest movement) between the humerus and the scapula. The humerus is a strong bone and its angulation allows for shock absorption. The shoulder movement is mainly flexion and extension, with some rotation, abduction and adduction.

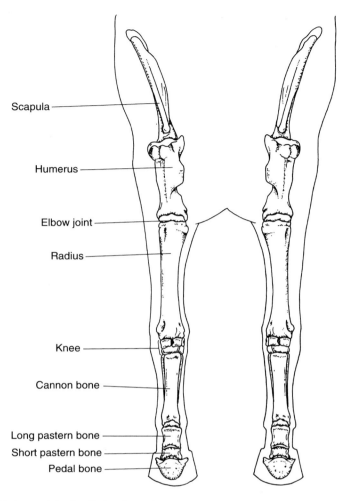

Fig. 3.3   Skeleton of the forelimb – front view

Radius and ulna

The radius and ulna are equivalent to the bones of the human lower arm but, unlike the human, they are fused together to prevent the horse's foreleg from twisting. The ulna is very small except for the olecranon process, which forms part of the elbow. The elbow is a ginglymus joint between the humerus, radius and ulna, and allows movement in one direction only.

Knee (carpus) (Figs 3.5, 3.6)

The knee or carpus is equivalent to the human wrist and consists of seven or eight small carpal bones arranged in two rows, one above the other.

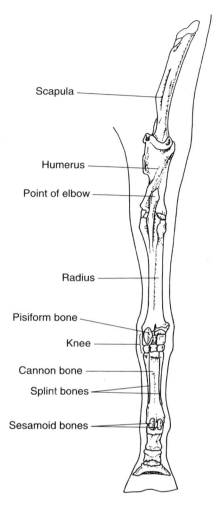

Scapula

Humerus

Point of elbow

Radius

Pisiform bone

Knee

Cannon bone

Splint bones

Sesamoid bones

Fig. 3.4   Skeleton of the forelimb – rear view

- Upper row – radial, intermediate and ulna carpals with the accessory carpal or pisiform bone, which does not bear weight, at the back
- Lower row – first, second, third and fourth carpals.

The joint is designed to absorb shock. It is a hinge (ginglymus) joint because it only moves in one direction, i.e. flexion and extension; as the knee flexes, the hoof moves towards the elbow. There is no lateral or rotational movement.

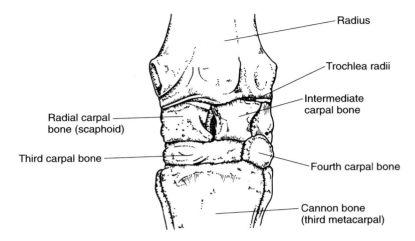

Radius

Trochlea radii

Intermediate carpal bone

Radial carpal bone (scaphoid)

Third carpal bone

Fourth carpal bone

Cannon bone (third metacarpal)

Fig. 3.5   Knee – front view

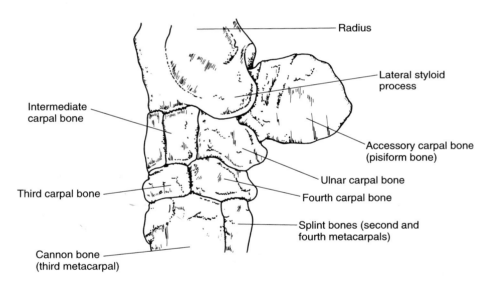

Radius

Lateral styloid process

Intermediate carpal bone

Accessory carpal bone (pisiform bone)

Ulnar carpal bone

Third carpal bone

Fourth carpal bone

Splint bones (second and fourth metacarpals)

Cannon bone (third metacarpal)

Fig. 3.6   Knee – side view

Conformation (Fig. 3.7)

The horse's limbs are not ideally suited to long-term, repeated and strenuous work, but an individual's conformation will make that horse less or more likely to stay sound throughout an athletic career. This means that optimal conformation of the forelimbs is particularly important in performance horses and that a basic knowledge of conformation is very useful when purchasing a horse.

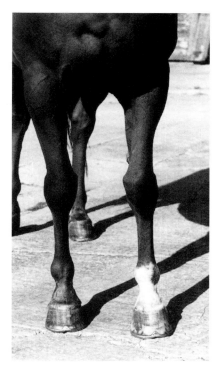

Fig. 3.7 Forelimb conformation

Differences between breeds

Conformational differences exist between the lighter types of horse such as the Arab and Thoroughbred, and the heavier draught horses such as the Shire. Draught horses have more 'bone': the circumference of the cannon bone just below the knee is greater than in lighter horses, this being associated with their superior weight-carrying capacity. Draught horses also tend to be more upright though the shoulder and the pastern, giving them a short, jarring stride, while the sloping shoulder and pastern of the Thoroughbred give a longer, springy stride.

Ideal conformation

Shoulder

The horse should have a good sloping shoulder so that there is 'plenty in front of the rider' and the saddle sits in a comfortable position. A long, correctly angulated scapula will also allow for a longer stride length. Traditionally the ideal shoulder has a 45° slope to the horizontal with a similar hoof–pastern angle. This enables concussive forces to be absorbed equally by all components of the limb. In practice, as long as the shoulder is flat and long enough to ensure a good stride length, it does not matter if it is a little upright.

The humerus is very strong and its angulation, which should be about 60° to the horizontal, allows for shock absorption. The slope of the shoulder should balance the pelvis and hip articulation; it is no good if the forehand has extravagant movement that the hind limbs cannot match.

Elbow

The elbow should be 'free' and allow a fist to be placed between it and the ribs. A 'tied-in' elbow limits stride length. The point of the elbow should be in the same plane as the point of the shoulder, so that it does not turn in or out. The measurement from the withers to the point of the elbow should be about the same as from the point of the elbow to the ground, ensuring adequate depth of chest.

Forelimb

The forearm should be long and well muscled, and the cannon bone should be short with adequate flat bone. Seen from the side and front the forelimbs should be straight. From the front, a plumb-line dropped from the point of shoulder should bisect the limb and hoof. This shows that the bones are arranged in a column, directly on top of each other, giving strength and ensuring that concussive forces spread evenly up the limb. The space between the front feet when the horse is standing square should be large enough to accommodate another foot. The knee should be flat and broad at the front with good depth. Common faults include the following:

- Over at the knee – the knee appears to be slightly flexed
- Back at the knee – the front of the leg appears concave
- Tied in below the knee – there is less bone below the knee than there is lower down the leg
- Calf knees – shallow from front to back
- Offset cannon bones – the bones are not placed directly below the knee in a straight line.

The fetlock joints should be well defined and bony rather than puffy.

Seen from the side, a line dropped from the midpoint of the scapula should run down in front of the forelimb and pass down through the middle of the hoof. If this is difficult to visualise, it may be easier to locate the small projection or tuber on the scapula that lies a little above the mid point. A line dropped from here should pass down through the elbow joint, the knee and the fetlock and hit the ground just behind the heels. In addition, a line dropped from the elbow should run vertically down the back of the leg.

Feet

The shape and proportions of the feet should be suitable for the limb, a pair and 'in balance'.

Hoof balance

- A vertical axis drawn through the centre of the cannon bone should bisect the hoof into two equal halves
- A line running across the top of the coronary band should be horizontal, showing that the hoof wall is at the same angle on both sides
- The wall should not flare out or run under
- The frog should bisect the foot exactly
- The hoof should be the same shape and size on either side of the frog
- The hoof–pastern axis (HPA) should be in alignment. The ideal hoof angle is 45–50° in front and 50–55° for the hind feet. In practice, depending on the individual horse's conformation, the angles tend to be more upright than this
- The angle of the hoof wall at the toe should be the same as at the heel
- The hoof should land level and slightly heel first.

Musculature (Figs 1.4, 3.8, 3.9, 5.4, 5.5)

Trapezius

The trapezius muscle is a flattened triangular sheet of superficial muscle consisting of long muscle fibres which run more or less parallel to its long axis. It is divided into the thoracic and cervical parts and is attached to the bones by sheet-like tendons. The cervical part attaches to the cervical vertebrae and the scapula, whilst the thoracic part originates on the thoracic vertebrae and inserts onto the scapula; it draws the scapula up and back to lift the shoulder, and is able to produce a large movement because its component muscle fibres are long.

Rhomboideus

The rhomboideus lies underneath the trapezius and ties the scapula into the sides of the spinous processes of the thoracic vertebrae and the nuchal ligament. It lifts the shoulder up and forwards.

Deltoid

The deltoid muscle arises from the scapula spine. It runs down to meet the brachiocephalicus muscle before inserting into the humerus. It flexes the shoulder joint to move the forelimb away from the body, i.e. abduct it.

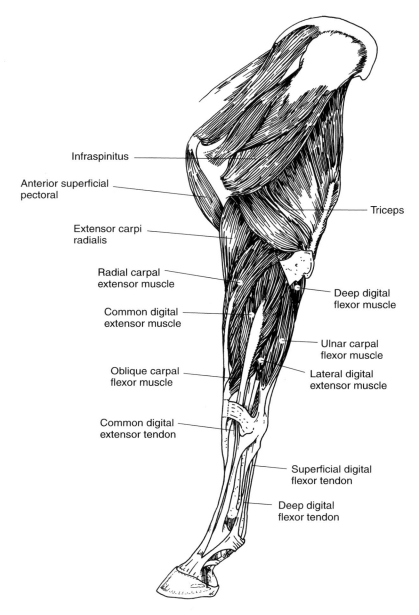

Infraspinitus

Anterior superficial
pectoral

Extensor carpi
radialis

Radial carpal
extensor muscle

Common digital
extensor muscle

Oblique carpal
flexor muscle

Common digital
extensor tendon

Triceps

Deep digital
flexor muscle

Ulnar carpal
flexor muscle

Lateral digital
extensor muscle

Superficial digital
flexor tendon

Deep digital
flexor tendon

Fig. 3.8 Muscles of the forelimb – side view

Triceps

The triceps is made up of three muscles running from the scapula to the point of the elbow. The long head of the triceps originates on the scapula; it flexes the shoulder and extends the elbow joint. The lateral and medial heads are shorter and originate on the humerus, acting to extend the elbow joint.

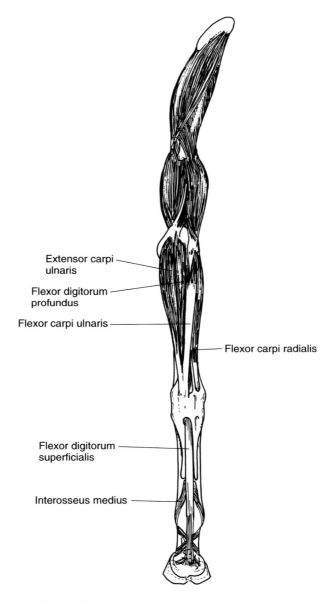

Extensor carpi
ulnaris

Flexor digitorum
profundus

Flexor carpi ulnaris

Flexor carpi radialis

Flexor digitorum
superficialis

Interosseus medius

Fig. 3.9 Muscles of the forelimb – rear view

Latissimus dorsi

The latissimus dorsi lies behind the shoulder. It originates on the thoracic and lumbar vertebrae and attaches to the rear of the humerus. Hence it covers the side and top of the chest. It flexes the shoulder joint and draws the scapula down and back, taking the forelimb back. Thus when the foot is on the ground, contraction of the latissimus dorsi moves the body forwards over the limb. Like the trapezius, it is a large flat sheet made up of many muscle fibres running parallel to its long axis and is attached to bones by sheet-like tendons. Because its constituent muscle fibres are long, it produces a large movement when it contracts.

Pectoral muscles

The pectoral muscles pass from the sternum to the humerus, forming a triangular sheet. The superficial pectorals are easily seen on the front of the chest. They support the humerus and pull it back to bring the limb back towards the body, i.e. adduct it.

Supraspinatus

The supraspinitus muscle originates in front of the scapula spines and attaches to the humerus. Its role is to advance the limb.

Infraspinatus

The infraspinitus muscle originates behind the ridge of the scapula spine and attaches to the humerus. It moves the forearm away from the body and allows it to rotate outwards.

Digital extensors

These form a mass of muscle at the front of the foreleg, originating on the humerus and radius and attaching to the long pastern, short pastern and pedal bones via the digital extensor tendons. Their role is to carry the limb and foot forwards.

Digital flexors

The digital flexor muscles originate on the humerus and the point of the elbow; they attach to the short pastern and pedal bone. Their role is to flex the knee, fetlock and foot.

The lower limb (Fig. 3.10)

During the course of evolution the lower limb lengthened below the knee and hock and the digits reduced in number, leaving just the middle digit and two vestigial lateral digits (the splint bones). This means that the horse's knee is equivalent to the human wrist and the metacarpal bones (cannon and splint bones) are equivalent to those between the human wrist and the knuckles. The first, second and third phalangeal bones (long pastern, short pastern and pedal bones) are equivalent to the three bones

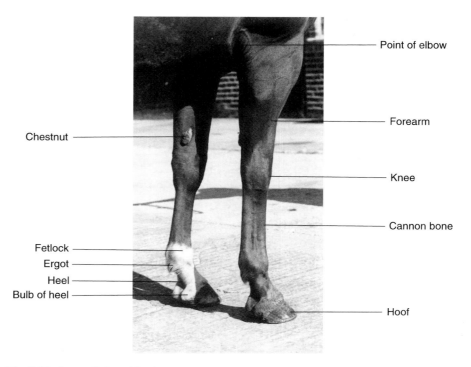

Point of elbow

Forearm

Knee

Cannon bone

Chestnut

Fetlock
Ergot
Heel
Bulb of heel

Hoof

Fig. 3.10 Lower limb – side view

of the human middle finger: in effect, the horse stands on the equivalent of the tip of the human middle finger. To keep the limb light, there are no muscles below the knee; therefore the tendons of the lower leg also had to lengthen to transmit the contractions of muscles higher up the limb to this area.

Skeleton of the lower limb (Figs 3.11, 3.12)

Metacarpal (cannon and splint) bones
There are three metacarpal bones, two of which (the splint bones) have regressed over time; the third metacarpal is the weight-bearing cannon bone. The weight-carrying capacity of the horse is indicated by the amount of 'bone' that it has, i.e. by the circumference of the cannon bone just below the knee.

Fetlock joint
The fetlock is the joint between the cannon bone, long pastern bone and two proximal sesamoid bones. It is a hinge (ginglymus) joint with a wide range of movement; its role is to transfer forces up and down the limb. The proximal sesamoid bones lie on either side at the back of the fetlock,

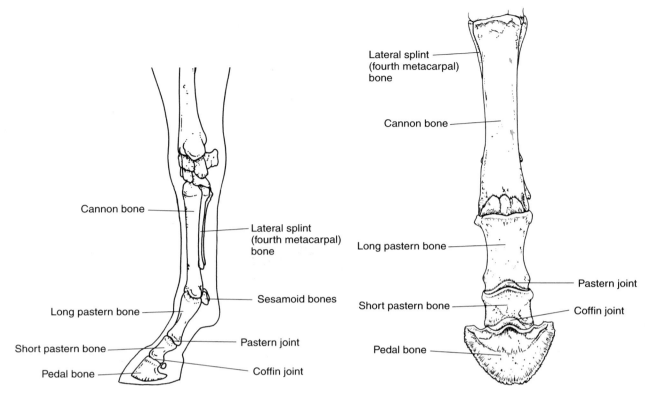

Fig. 3.11   Skeleton of the lower limb – side view

Fig. 3.12   Skeleton of the lower limb – front view

behind the lower end of the cannon bone. Each sesamoid bone is shaped like a three-sided pyramid and is moulded to the cannon bone.

Pastern
The pastern is the area between the lower end of the fetlock and the foot. It is made up of the first and second pastern bones. The long pastern, short pastern and pedal bone are also known as the phalanges. The tendons from the muscles of the forearm attach to these bones and their angle should be the same as the angle of the shoulder, 45°.

Pastern joint
The pastern joint occurs between the long and short pastern bones. It is also a ginglymus joint and is the least moveable of the joints in the area.

Sesamoid bones
The proximal sesamoid bones are known simply as the sesamoids and are situated at the back of the fetlock joint. The distal sesamoid bone or

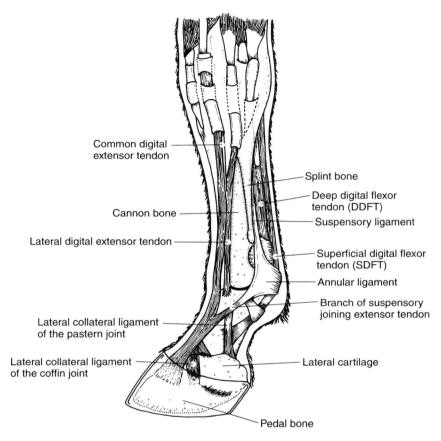

Common digital
extensor tendon

Cannon bone

Lateral digital extensor tendon

Lateral collateral ligament
of the pastern joint

Lateral collateral ligament
of the coffin joint

Splint bone

Deep digital flexor
tendon (DDFT)

Suspensory ligament

Superficial digital flexor
tendon (SDFT)

Annular ligament

Branch of suspensory
joining extensor tendon

Lateral cartilage

Pedal bone

Fig. 3.13   Tendons and ligaments of the lower limb

navicular bone is found at the rear of the coffin joint in the hoof capsule. The sesamoid bones act as pulleys, enabling the tendons to exert their pull on the phalanges.

Coffin joint

The second pastern bone forms the coffin joint with the pedal and navicular bones within the hoof. It is a ginglymus joint with limited flexion and extension, and limited rotation on manual movement.

Tendons and ligaments of the lower limb (Figs 3.13–3.15)

Tendons are strong extensions of a muscle that connect that muscle to bone. They are relatively inelastic because their role is to pull the skeleton in response to muscle contraction. The tendons and muscles work together to allow the horse to move.

Tendons run from the muscles of the horse's foreleg in grooves of the

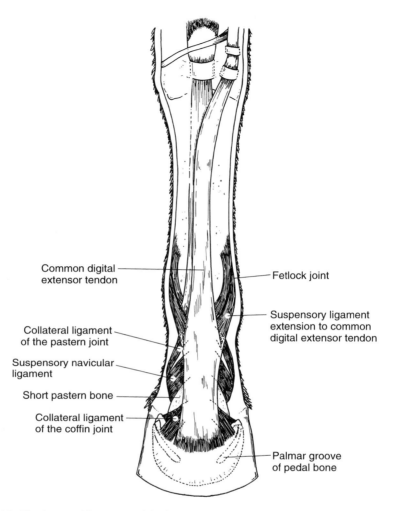

Common digital
extensor tendon

Fetlock joint

Suspensory ligament
extension to common
digital extensor tendon

Collateral ligament
of the pastern joint

Suspensory navicular
ligament

Short pastern bone

Collateral ligament
of the coffin joint

Palmar groove
of pedal bone

Fig. 3.14   Tendons and ligaments of the lower limb – front view

bone across the knee and fetlock. They are held in position by canals of
connective tissue called the annular ligaments: these ligaments encircle
the tendons at the top and bottom to keep them correctly aligned. To
prevent friction as the tendon moves, it is surrounded by a tendon sheath.
The tendon sheath has an outer layer attached to the lining of the canal
and an inner structure attached to the surface of the tendon. Synovial fluid
is secreted between these two layers to allow the surfaces to run smoothly
over one another.

   The tendon itself consists of fibres running along its entire length. The
fibres are made up of densely packed bundles of collagen, arranged
parallel to each other. These fibres are 'crimped': they are not straight but
bent in a regular zig-zag pattern, giving the tendon the ability to increase
slightly in length. As the muscle contracts and pulls on the tendon, the

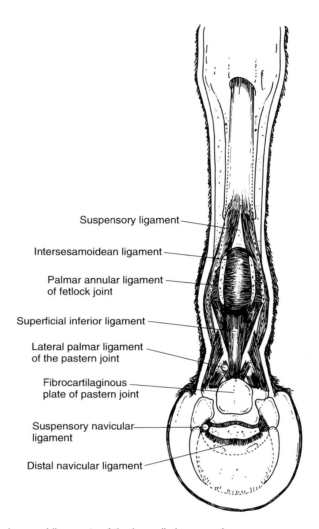

Suspensory ligament

Intersesamoidean ligament

Palmar annular ligament
of fetlock joint

Superficial inferior ligament

Lateral palmar ligament
of the pastern joint

Fibrocartilaginous
plate of pastern joint

Suspensory navicular
ligament

Distal navicular ligament

Fig. 3.15 Tendons and ligaments of the lower limb – rear view

crimp straightens before the tendon exerts pull on the bone to which it is attached. When the load is removed the crimp returns. This system helps to prevent damage to the tendon.

Collagen is a type of protein and is continuously being replaced. There are several types of collagen in the body; healthy tendons are made up of type I collagen, which is relatively elastic. If the tendon is damaged the repair tissue is initially made up of less resilient type III collagen. Additionally the new collagen is laid down haphazardly, not in parallel lines. Both factors result in the healing tendon being highly susceptible to further injury.

The fetlock is supported at the back by the superficial and deep flexor tendons, the suspensory apparatus and the annular ligament, and does

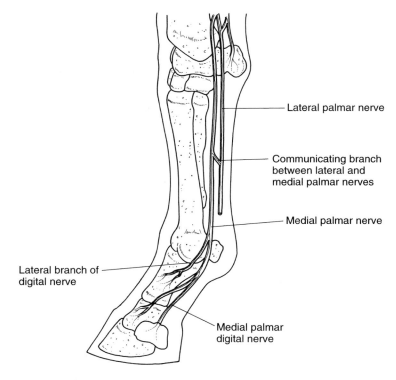

Lateral palmar nerve

Communicating branch
between lateral and
medial palmar nerves

Medial palmar nerve

Lateral branch of
digital nerve

Medial palmar
digital nerve

Fig. 3.16   Nerves of the lower forelimb

not experience any direct forces during movement. At the back of the
fetlock the superficial flexor tendon forms a ring through which the
deep flexor tendon moves. The tendons are further bound by the annular
ligament of the fetlock joint. The two proximal sesamoids act as a pulley
over which the deep flexor tendon runs, and strong ligaments bind the
sesamoids to the suspensory apparatus. The foot and pastern should be
positioned so that a line drawn along the front surface of each is not
broken either forwards or backwards. Figures 3.14 and 3.15 show the
insertions of the tendons and ligaments of the lower limb.

Nerves of the lower limb (Fig. 3.16)

Forelimb nerves originate from the brachial plexus, a network of branches
from the last three cervical and the first two thoracic spinal nerves. Nerves
accompany the arteries down the leg. Both palmar nerves branch dorsally
into the front of the pastern, the remainder of the nerves penetrating the
foot and supplying the sensitive tissues of the hoof.

The veterinary procedure known as 'denerving' refers to the surgical
cutting of the palmar or plantar digital nerve to relieve chronic pain
permanently. A nerve block consists of injections of local anaesthetic

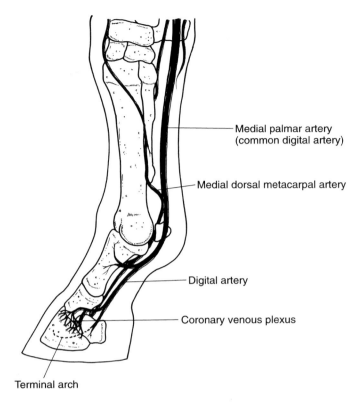

Medial palmar artery
(common digital artery)

Medial dorsal metacarpal artery

Digital artery

Coronary venous plexus

Terminal arch

Fig. 3.17   Blood supply of lower forelimb

at strategic points into the nerves of the lower limb to locate the site of pain.

Blood supply of the lower limb (Fig. 3.17)

Blood reaching the hoof flows primarily through a sequence of arteries, the axillary, brachial, median, medial palmar, and medial and lateral digital. The two digital arteries meet to form the terminal arch within the solar canal of the pedal bone, nourishing sensitive structures within the hoof.

Veins run alongside the arteries draining from a coronary venous plexus which circles the upper part of the foot. Blood is then forced back up towards the heart through the veins in the leg. Concussive pressure from the horse's foot on the venous complexes pushes blood back up the leg against gravity.

Foot and hoof (Figs 3.18, 3.19)

The foot of the horse is equivalent to the human middle finger, consisting of three bones, the long pastern, short pastern and pedal bone. These

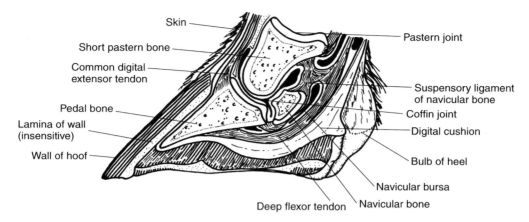

Skin
Short pastern bone
Common digital extensor tendon
Pedal bone
Lamina of wall (insensitive)
Wall of hoof
Pastern joint
Suspensory ligament of navicular bone
Coffin joint
Digital cushion
Bulb of heel
Navicular bursa
Navicular bone
Deep flexor tendon

Fig. 3.18 Cross-section of the foot

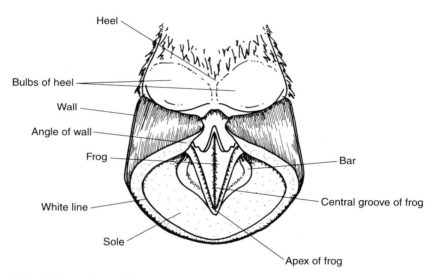

Heel
Bulbs of heel
Wall
Angle of wall
Frog
White line
Sole
Bar
Central groove of frog
Apex of frog

Fig. 3.19 Undersurface of the foot

bones articulate to give the fetlock, pastern and coffin joints. The hoof surrounds the pedal bone, the navicular bone and part of the short pastern bone.

The horse's hoof is a highly specialised structure designed to

- Resist wear and tear
- Support the horse's body weight
- Absorb concussion.

The external hoof is a continuation of modified skin, similar to claws and horns in other animals, which encloses the sensitive structures within.

Hoof wall

The wall is produced by and grows down from the coronary band. It consists of dense horn and is divided into the toe, quarters and heels. At the heels the wall is reflected back, inwards and forwards to form the bars of the hoof.

Periople

The wall is covered by a thin layer of epidermis called the periople, which originates from a rim of soft grey horn at the coronary band.

Sole

The sole is crescent shaped and concave so that it arches over the ground, protecting sensitive structures within the foot.

Frog

The frog is a wedge of soft, elastic horn situated between the hoof bars. It blends with the bulbs of heels on each side. The frog has a central groove dividing it into two crura. The frog acts as a shock absorber, assists circulation and aids grip. When the frog hits the ground it is compressed and expands sideways, so putting pressure on the digital cushion which, in turn, squeezes the lateral cartilages and wall of the foot so that the wall expands.

Stay apparatus of the forelimb (Fig. 3.20)

Horses may rest for long periods of time in a standing position which has the advantage of allowing a faster get-away should predators attack. Horses can sleep in the standing position due to a system of muscles and ligaments that 'lock' the main joints into position without expending a lot of energy so that the muscles do not become fatigued. This arrangement is much the same in both the forelimbs and hind limbs. Normally both forelimbs are locked whilst one hind limb is relaxed or rested.

The stay apparatus in the forelimbs includes

- The suspensory ligament
- The deep digital flexor tendon with the deep digital flexor muscle running from the elbow to the back of the pedal bone
- The carpal check ligament which joins the deep digital flexor tendon to the cannon bone
- The superficial digital flexor tendon and muscle from the elbow to the short pastern bone
- The radial check ligament.

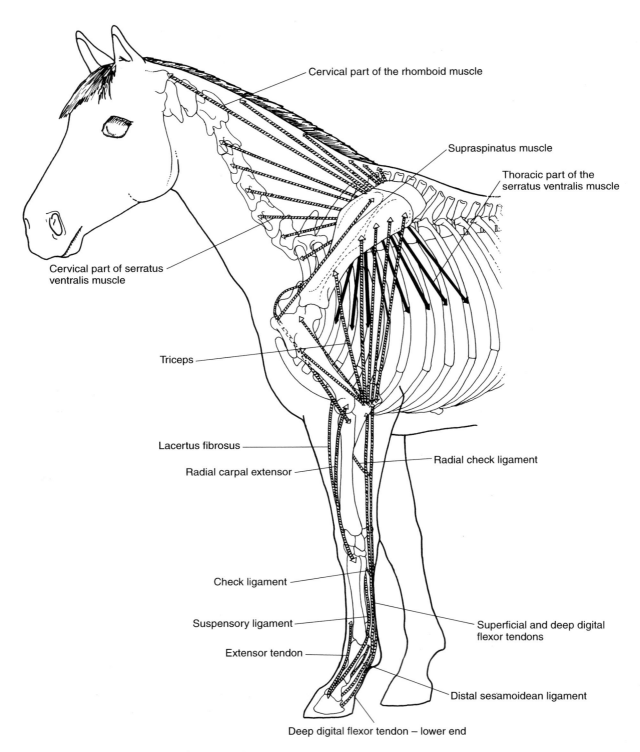

Cervical part of the rhomboid muscle

Supraspinatus muscle

Thoracic part of the
serratus ventralis muscle

Cervical part of serratus
ventralis muscle

Triceps

Lacertus fibrosus

Radial carpal extensor

Radial check ligament

Check ligament

Suspensory ligament

Extensor tendon

Superficial and deep digital
flexor tendons

Distal sesamoidean ligament

Deep digital flexor tendon – lower end

Fig. 3.20 Stay apparatus of the forelimb

Check ligaments

The superficial digital flexor tendon of the forelimb has a check ligament that links into the radius of the forearm. The ligament prevents the tendon being pulled too far down when the fetlock is weight-bearing and so helps to prevent the fetlock collapsing onto the ground. The carpal check ligament of the deep digital flexor tendon links to the carpal bones of the knee.

Suspensory ligament

The suspensory ligament attaches to the top of the knee and runs down the back of the leg between the cannon bone and the flexor tendons. Just above the fetlock joint it divides in two, with each branch attaching to one of the two sesamoid bones, and then continues forward to join the extensor tendon at the front of the pastern.

Suspension of the fetlock

The suspensory ligament provides a link between the extensor and flexor systems, literally suspending the fetlock joint. When the body weight of the horse presses down on the fetlock joint, the suspensory ligament tightens, followed by the superficial flexor and deep digital flexor tendons. Higher in the forelimb, the elbow is prevented from flexing which, in turn, means that the biceps brachii muscle, extending from the shoulderblade to the forearm, can stop the shoulder from flexing. The knee is prevented from buckling forwards by the lacertus fibrosus tendon.

Care of the horse's legs

It is important to be able to identify the structures of the lower leg in the healthy horse so that the first signs of over-use or lameness can be located and acted upon before permanent damage is done. The cannon and the two splint bones can be easily felt under the skin. The splint bone is sometimes mistaken for the suspensory ligament; however, the splint bones lie very close to the cannon bone and each one ends in an obvious small lump about three-quarters of the way down the cannon bone. Individual horses will have varying amounts of warmth and thickness in the lower leg and the forelegs may differ from the hind legs. The normal condition for each individual horse should be known.

Tendons and ligaments of the lower leg

Healthy tendons are made of relatively elastic type I collagen, whereas after damage the repair tissue is made up of less resilient type III collagen laid down haphazardly, not in parallel lines. Both these factors mean that during healing a tendon is very susceptible to further injury. Horses recovering from tendon injury need:

- Box rest until sound in walk
- Physiotherapy and/or veterinary intervention
- Controlled walking to help align the new collagen correctly
- Time for the new collagen to be replaced by stronger type I collagen, i.e. a minimum period of 6 months
- A carefully controlled re-introduction to work.

It is important to remember that horses will be sound before full healing has taken place and this may lead to them being brought back into work too soon.

Minimising the risk of tendon injury

- Carry out regular and correct shoeing to prevent long toe – low heel conformation
- Do not continue to work a fatigued horse
- Do not work horses on uneven or poor ground
- Do not ignore the early warning signs – often there is a re-occurring slight injury before the horse 'breaks down'. Watch out for any mild heat and swelling even if the horse is sound.

Chapter 4

The hind limb

Introduction

The hind limb provides the propulsion for the horse to move forwards, often at great speed. The athletic horse has not only to move at speed, but also to perform sharp turns and sudden stops which require balance and co-ordination.

The hindquarters

Equine sports such as show jumping, dressage and polo, rely on the transfer of the centre of gravity towards the hindquarters which are highly muscular and must be well developed to give great power and propulsion. The upper hind limb is different anatomically from the forelimb, but is the same below the hock.

The hindquarters of the horse are characteristically rounded due to the huge muscles of this area. The muscles in this mass originate on the horse's pelvis, extending from the sacral and coccygeal vertebrae to the stifle; there are also complex attachments to the inner and outer surfaces of the tibia.

Alignment (Fig. 4.1)

If standing at the side of the horse, a plumb line dropped from the point of the buttock to the point of the hock, should fall in alignment with the back of the tendons to the fetlock.

The stifle is turned out slightly, allowing the horse to move forwards freely, this may result in the foot being slightly toe-out.

The skeleton (Fig. 4.2)

The hind limb consists of the following bones:

- Its half of the pelvis
- Femur

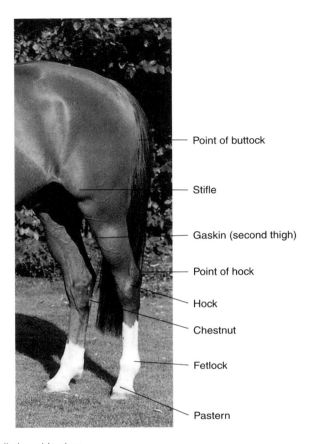

Point of buttock

Stifle

Gaskin (second thigh)

Point of hock

Hock

Chestnut

Fetlock

Pastern

Fig. 4.1 Hind limb – side view

- Tibia and fibula
- Tarsal bones of the hock
- Three metacarpals (cannon and splint bones)
- Long pastern (first phalanx)
- Short pastern (second phalanx)
- Pedal bone (third phalanx)
- Two sesamoid bones
- Navicular bone (also a type of sesamoid bone).

Pelvic girdle (Fig. 4.3)

The pelvic girdle consists of the sacrum comprising fused sacral vertebrae, two pelvic bones, and the first three coccygeal vertebrae. Each pelvic bone (os coxae) is made up of three flat bones, the ilium, pubis and ischium, which are fused into one. All three bones meet at the acetabulum which articulates with the head of the femur to form the hip joint.

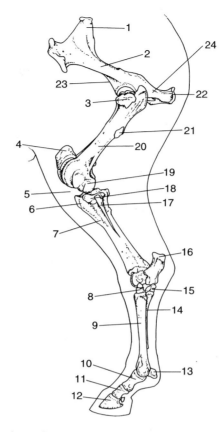

1 Tuber sacrale (point of croup)
2 Ilium
3 Cranial part of trochanter of femur
4 Patella
5 Stifle
6 Tibial crest
7 Tibia
8 Third tarsal bone
9 Cannon bone
10 Long pastern bone
11 Short pastern bone
12 Pedal bone

13 Proximal sesamoid bone
14 Splint bone
15 Fourth tarsal bone
16 Tuber calcis (point of hock)
17 Fibula
18 Lateral condyle of tibia
19 Lateral condyle of femur
20 Femur
21 Third trochanter of femur
22 Tuber ischii (point of buttock)
23 Pubis
24 Ischium

Fig. 4.2 Skeleton of the hind limb – side view

Ilium

The ilium is the largest of the three bones making up the os coxae; its outermost angle is seen as the point of the hip or tuber coxae, and the internal angles (tuber sacrale) of the two ilia together form the croup at the highest point of the hindquarters immediately behind the loins. The ilium attaches to the sacrum at the sacroiliac joint, a combined synovial and

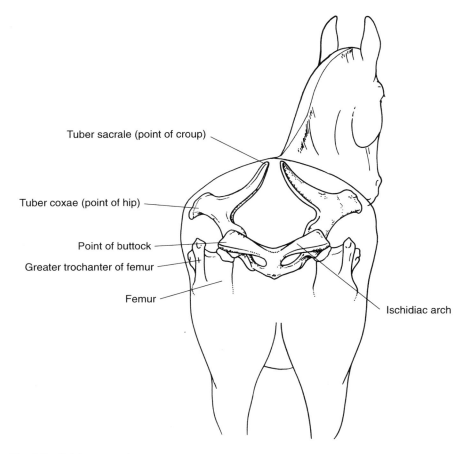

Fig. 4.3   Pelvis – rear view

fibrocartilagenous joint which is supported by ventral, dorsal and lateral sacroiliac ligaments (see Chapter 6).

Pubis
This bone forms the front of the pelvic floor; the right and left pubis meet at the pelvic symphysis which ossifies with age.

Ischium
This bone forms the rear part of the pelvis; its thickened end is known as the tuber ischii and forms the point of the buttock.

Femur (Figs 4.4–4.6)

The femur is a very strong bone between the hip joint and the stifle joint and is adapted for the attachment of the muscles of the hindquarter.

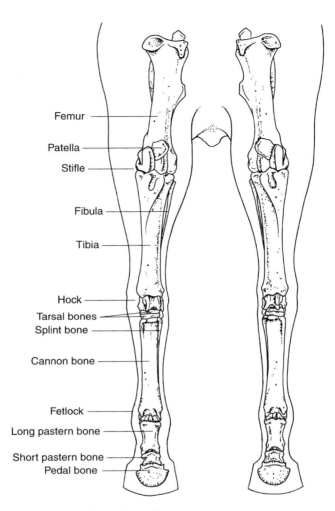

Femur
Patella
Stifle
Fibula
Tibia
Hock
Tarsal bones
Splint bone
Cannon bone
Fetlock
Long pastern bone
Short pastern bone
Pedal bone

Fig. 4.4   Skeleton of the hind limb – front view

Tarsal bones

The hock or tarsus consists of six or seven short, flat tarsal bones arranged in three rows. In the upper row are the talus and calcaneus: in the middle row is the central tarsus and below that the fused first and second tarsal and the third tarsal. The fourth tarsal occupies both the middle and lower row.

Patella

The patella is a sesamoid bone associated with the stifle and is the equivalent of the human kneecap.

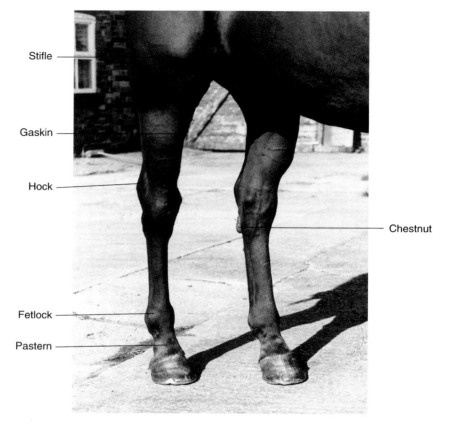

Stifle

Gaskin

Hock

Chestnut

Fetlock

Pastern

Fig. 4.5 Hind limb – front view

Point of hock

The long bony process, the tuber calcis of the calcaneus, gives rise to the point of the hock and guides the Achilles tendon of the gastrocnemius muscle over the hock, allowing tremendous leverage.

Tibia

The tibia is a long bone running down and back between the stifle and the hock joints. The upper end provides attachment for the muscles acting on the hock and lower limb. The horse's fibula is so reduced in size as to be practically vestigial.

Lower limb (Fig. 4.7)

Below the hock the anatomical arrangement is the same as in the forelimb.

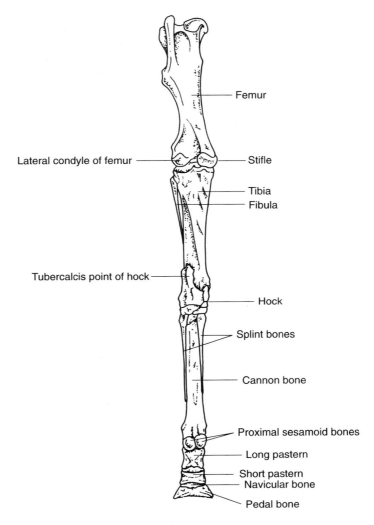

Fig. 4.6 Skeleton of the hind limb – rear view

Joints of the hind limb

Hip

The hip joint is deep in the hindquarter of the horse and is most easily seen when the hind leg is flexed. It is the joint between the pelvis and the femur and is capable of a wide range of movement. It protects the internal organs and acts as a site for muscle attachment to allow the efficient transfer of force to the spine.

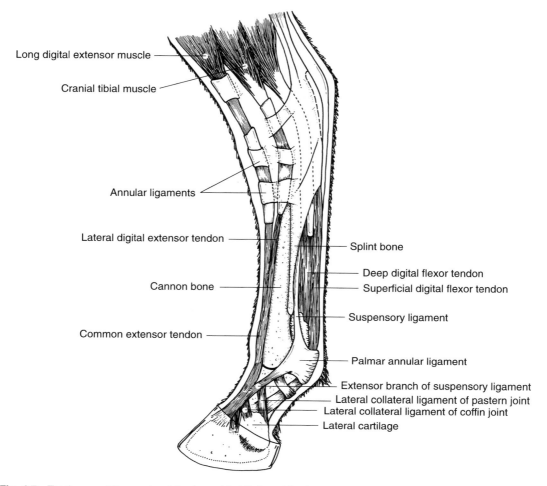

Long digital extensor muscle

Cranial tibial muscle

Annular ligaments

Lateral digital extensor tendon

Cannon bone

Common extensor tendon

Splint bone

Deep digital flexor tendon

Superficial digital flexor tendon

Suspensory ligament

Palmar annular ligament

Extensor branch of suspensory ligament

Lateral collateral ligament of pastern joint

Lateral collateral ligament of coffin joint

Lateral cartilage

Fig. 4.7   Tendons and ligaments of the lower hind limb – side view

Stifle (Fig. 4.8)

The stifle joint is the largest in the horse's body. One of its main functions is to cause the limb to become rigid when the foot is placed on the ground. This is achieved by contraction of the muscles inserted into the patella. In upward fixation of the patella where no flexion of the stifle and hock can occur, the lower limb joints such as the coffin, pastern and fetlock can still be flexed. The semiflexed position of the stifle joint helps it to act as a shock absorber and reduce the effects of concussion.

Hock (Figs 4.9–4.12)

The hock joint, although composed of numerous bones, has a smaller amount of movement than the knee joint. The partial flexion of the hock joint at all times helps it to absorb shock and reduce the effects of concussion.

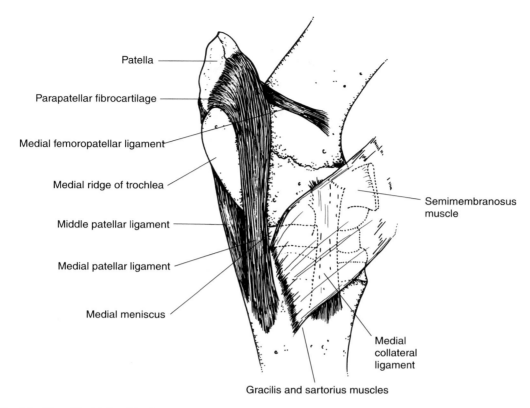

Patella

Parapatellar fibrocartilage

Medial femoropatellar ligament

Medial ridge of trochlea

Middle patellar ligament

Medial patellar ligament

Medial meniscus

Semimembranosus muscle

Medial collateral ligament

Gracilis and sartorius muscles

Fig. 4.8   The stifle joint – side view

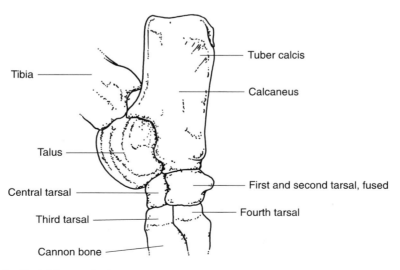

Tibia

Talus

Central tarsal

Third tarsal

Cannon bone

Tuber calcis

Calcaneus

First and second tarsal, fused

Fourth tarsal

Fig. 4.9   Hock joint – side view

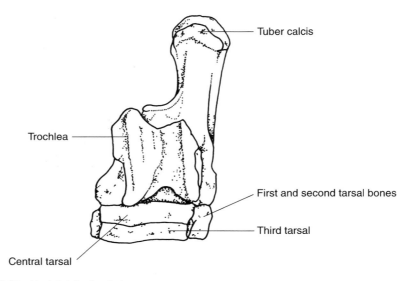

Tuber calcis

Trochlea

First and second tarsal bones

Third tarsal

Central tarsal

Fig. 4.10   Hock joint – front view

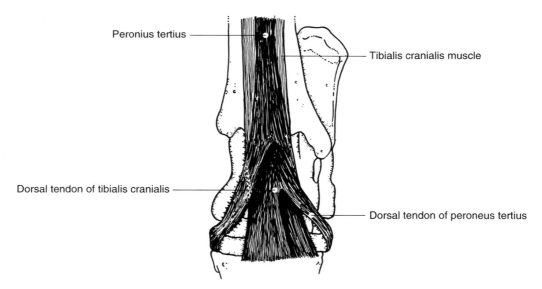

Peronius tertius

Tibialis cranialis muscle

Dorsal tendon of tibialis cranialis

Dorsal tendon of peroneus tertius

Fig. 4.11   Hock joint: insertion of flexors – front view

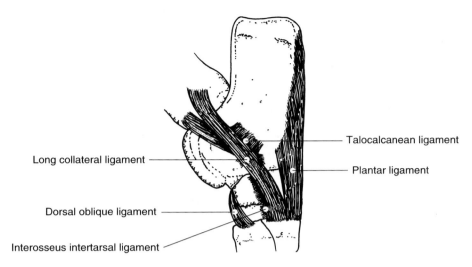

Talocalcanean ligament

Plantar ligament

Long collateral ligament

Dorsal oblique ligament

Interosseus intertarsal ligament

Fig. 4.12   Hock joint: insertion of flexors – side view

Muscles (Figs 4.13–4.15)

The hindquarters extend out and back from the point of croup and consist of a mass of muscle clothing the pelvis and femur and running down the thigh to the hock and lower leg.

Gluteal muscles

The gluteal muscles make up the bulk of the muscle mass that gives the hindquarters their characteristic rounded appearance. The gluteals arise from the shaft of the ilium and insert onto the femur. They act as strong hip extensors, which are involved in rearing, kicking and galloping.

Biceps femoris

The biceps femoris extends from the sacral and coccygeal vertebrae to attach to the femur and stifle joint. Its function is to extend and abduct the hind limb, i.e. propulsion, rearing and kicking.

Semitendinosus

The semitendinosus is a long muscle extending along the rear of the biceps femoris down the back of the thigh. The division between these two muscles is known as the poverty line and is clearly seen in thin or fit horses. This muscle originates in the pelvis and inserts onto the tibia. Its function is to extend the hip and hock and flex the stifle so that the limb

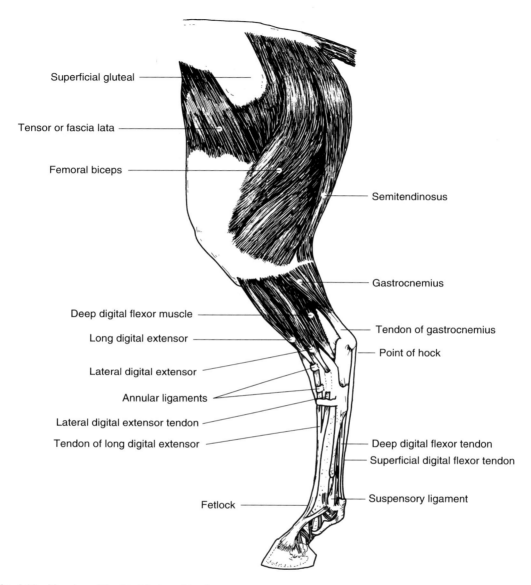

Fig. 4.13   Muscles of the hind limb – side view

is rotated inwards and provides propulsion. These muscles make up the hamstring group and are important in locomotion.

Semimembranosus

This muscle runs from the pelvis to the femur and stifle. When the limb is weight-bearing it extends the hip and stifle but when the limb is not supporting weight it adducts and rotates it inwards.

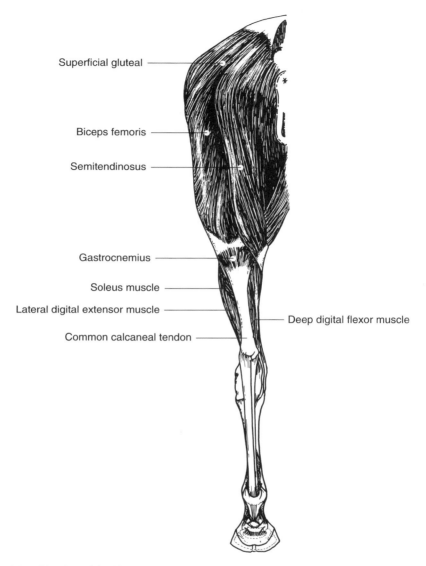

Fig. 4.14 Muscles of the hind limb – rear view

Digital extensors

The digital extensor muscles together with the hock flexor muscles make up the gaskin or second thigh. The digital extensors originate from the femur and insert onto the lower hind limb. They help to transmit movement to the toe via the tendons of the lower leg.

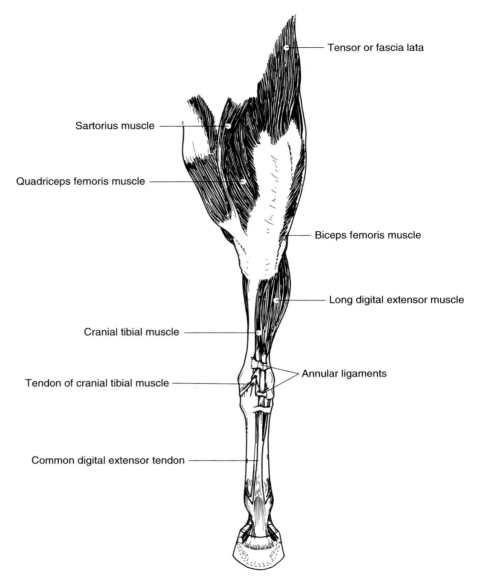

Tensor or fascia lata

Sartorius muscle

Quadriceps femoris muscle

Biceps femoris muscle

Long digital extensor muscle

Cranial tibial muscle

Annular ligaments

Tendon of cranial tibial muscle

Common digital extensor tendon

Fig. 4.15 Muscles of the hind limb – front view

Gastrocnemius

The gastrocnemius runs down the back of the limb ending in a large tendon. It is associated with the tendon of the deeper lying superficial flexor muscle; the combined tendon is palpable above the hock as the Achilles tendon. The tendon of the gastrocnemius attaches to the hock while the superficial flexor tendon runs over the hock and down the back of the limb to the foot. The function of the gastrocnemius is to move the hock.

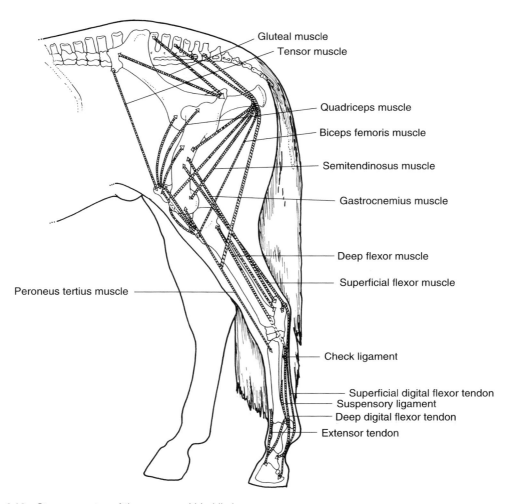

Fig. 4.16   Stay apparatus of the croup and hind limb

Stay apparatus of the hind limb (Fig. 4.16)

As discussed in Chapter 3, the stay apparatus allows the horse to rest in the standing position for long periods. It is a system of muscles and ligaments which is able to lock the joints into position. The stay apparatus of the lower hind limb is basically the same as that of the forelimb, but the superficial flexor tendon does not have an equivalent to the radial check ligament. The stay apparatus comprises the following:

- Fibrous sheet of serratus ventralis
- Tendon of biceps brachii
- Long head of triceps
- Lacertus fibrosus

- Deep digital flexor tendon
- Superficial digital flexor tendon
- Tensor fascia lata
- Gastrocnemius muscle
- Peroneus tertius muscle
- Deep digital flexor muscle
- Tarsal check ligament
- Superficial digital flexor muscle.

Stifle

The stifle cannot be moved without moving the hock through the action of the gastrocnemius and the peroneus tertius muscles.

Patella

The patella plays a vital role in the stay apparatus. It has a 'hook' which can lock over the inner trochlear ridge of the femur to fix the whole hind limb rigidly. If one joint of the leg is locked the others will not move readily, so when the horse wants to move it contracts the tensor fascia muscle which attaches to the patella thus slightly lifting and freeing the bone.

Hamstring muscles

The horse's weight is supported by a 'hammock' of hamstring muscles which runs over its buttocks.

Chapter 5

The chest

Introduction (Fig. 5.1)

The forelimbs are attached to the horse's body in an arrangement of muscles and ligaments known as the thoracic sling. The horse does not have a clavicle (collar bone) as does the human; there are no bones attaching the forelimbs to the body. This suspension of the thorax within the thoracic sling allows the horse some freedom to raise and lower the body, which allows much greater flexibility in movement. A side view of the chest is shown in Fig. 5.1; it contains the heart and lungs.

The skeleton (Fig. 5.2)

Ribs

Each thoracic vertebra articulates with a rib on either side. Therefore there are 18 pairs of ribs; these may be classified as sternal (true), asternal (false) or floating. The ribs form a bony cage to protect the lungs and heart; they are also an essential part of the breathing apparatus. The ribs contain spongy red bone marrow and are an important source of blood cells for the horse. In young horses, the ribs are quite soft, but as the horse gets older they become calcified and harden.

True ribs
There are eight pairs of sternal or 'true' ribs. Each rib head and tubercule forms a joint with each thoracic vertebra. The springiness of the rib is a property of its shaft or bony body. Each rib ends in a costal cartilage which is attached to the sternum.

Asternal or false ribs
The costal cartilages of ribs 9–18 are united by elastic tissue to form the costal arch. In turn, this is connected by fibrous tissue to the costal cartilage of rib eight.

Floating ribs
These do not reach the costal arch, ending freely in the musculature.

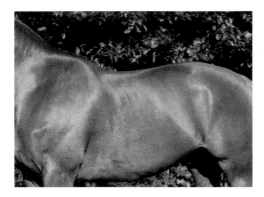

Fig. 5.1 Chest and ribs – side view

Sternum (Fig. 5.3)

The floor of the chest is formed by the sternum, which is held in position by the first eight pairs of ribs. The sternum is made up of a number of bones (stenebrae) held together by cartilage with which the sternal ends of the true ribs articulate, except for the first pair which articulate with the first sternebra (manubrium).

Xiphoid process
The rear end of the sternum is a flattened and heart shaped cartilagenous structure known as the xiphoid process to which muscle fibres of the diaphragm are attached.

Musculature (Figs 5.4, 5.5)

Intercostal muscles
Between the curved ribs lie the intercostal muscles which move them in a forward and outward direction helping the horse to breathe in.

Diaphragm
The diaphragm is a sheet of muscle and tendon separating the chest and abdominal cavities. Peripherally it is attached to the ventral surface of the lumbar vertebrae, the ribs and the sternum: the muscle fibres arise on these skeletal parts and radiate towards the tendinous centre. It projects forward into the chest cavity like a dome as far as the level of the seventh rib; this is almost opposite the olecranon in the standing horse.

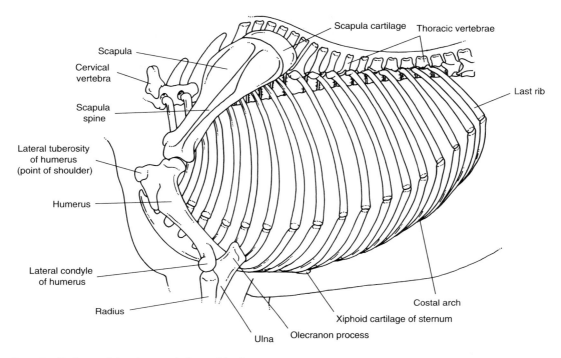

Fig. 5.2   Skeleton of the chest and ribs – side view

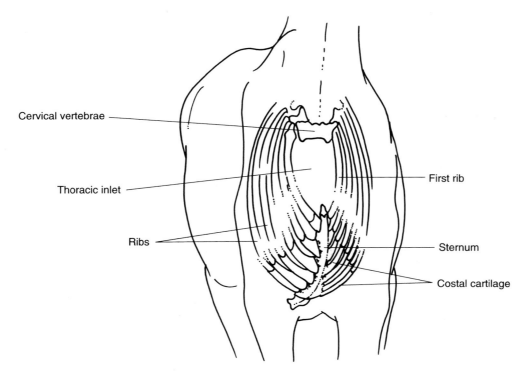

Fig. 5.3   Sternum – front view

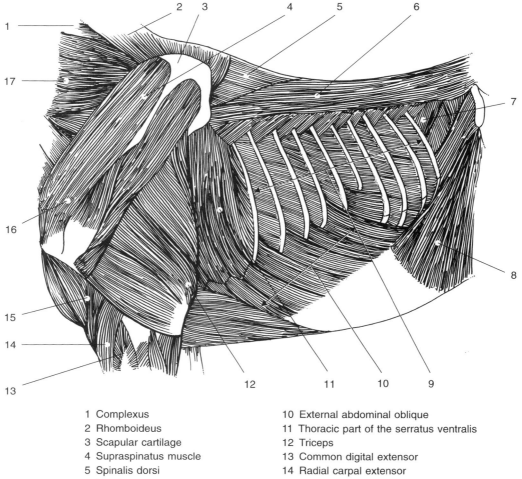

Fig. 5.4 Deep muscles of the chest – side view

1 Complexus	10 External abdominal oblique
2 Rhomboideus	11 Thoracic part of the serratus ventralis
3 Scapular cartilage	12 Triceps
4 Supraspinatus muscle	13 Common digital extensor
5 Spinalis dorsi	14 Radial carpal extensor
6 Longissimus dorsi	15 Biceps brachii muscle
7 Transverse abdominal oblique	16 Pectoral
8 Internal abdominal oblique	17 Cervical part of the serratus ventralis
9 External intercostal	

Serratus ventralis

The thoracic part of the serratus ventralis attaches to the lateral surfaces of the first nine ribs.

Nerves

Brachial plexus

The lateral part of the first rib has small grooves in which lie the vital nerves of the brachial plexus carrying both motor and sensory nervous

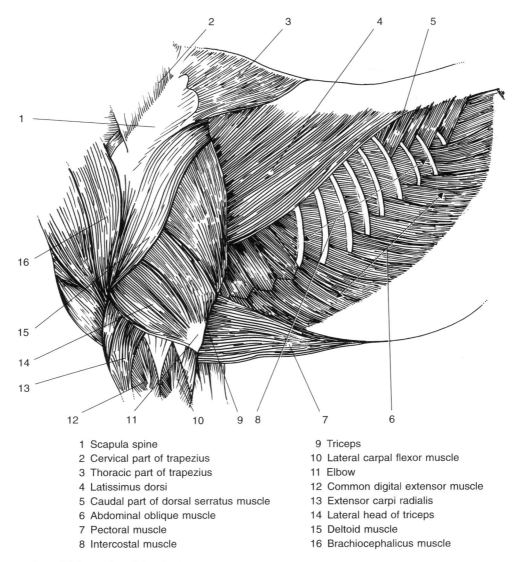

Fig. 5.5 Superficial muscles of the chest

1 Scapula spine
2 Cervical part of trapezius
3 Thoracic part of trapezius
4 Latissimus dorsi
5 Caudal part of dorsal serratus muscle
6 Abdominal oblique muscle
7 Pectoral muscle
8 Intercostal muscle

9 Triceps
10 Lateral carpal flexor muscle
11 Elbow
12 Common digital extensor muscle
13 Extensor carpi radialis
14 Lateral head of triceps
15 Deltoid muscle
16 Brachiocephalicus muscle

impulses to the forelimb. If this rib becomes damaged, for example by a fall, these nerves may also sustain damage, causing muscular paralysis.

Breathing

The horse requires a constant supply of oxygen to stay alive, and the process of breathing brings air containing oxygen into intimate contact with the blood in the lungs. The lungs occupy most of the horse's thoracic cavity, giving an enormous area for the transfer of oxygen into the blood.

Inhalation – breathing in

The horse draws air into its lungs through the action of the dome-shaped diaphragm and the external intercostal muscles. When the ribs are pulled forwards, upwards and outwards by contraction of the external intercostal muscles and the levatores costarum, the chest expands; simultaneously the diaphragm contracts, flattening the dome. Thus the 'box' in which the lungs are contained is enlarged and air is drawn in to fill the available space. As the diaphragm contracts the abdominal muscles relax, allowing the abdominal organs to move down and back. At rest the muscles of inhalation do not contract fully.

Exhalation – breathing out

The horse breathes out when the thorax decrease in size. Two groups of muscles effect breathing out: the abdominal muscles and the internal intercostal muscles. As the abdominal muscles contract, pressure is put on the abdominal organs which in turn press on the diaphragm and push it forwards into its resting (domed) position. The internal intercostal muscles rotate the ribs inwards and back to their resting position and the transverse thoracic muscles complete exhalation by compressing the thorax.

The muscles of exhalation do not contract fully when the horse is at rest. The recoil of the chest wall and the consequent collapse of the stretched lung tissue contribute significantly to reducing the volume of the thorax, so saving energy.

The average respiratory rate of the resting horse is between 8 and 16 breaths per minute. After strenuous exercise this can increase to up to 140 breaths per minute. During exercise the respiratory rate is linked to the horse's gait. At gallop there is locomotory–respiratory coupling and the stride rate is the same as the breathing rate. As the galloping horse lifts its forelimbs, the head is raised, external intercostal muscles and the diaphragm contract, abdominal muscles relax and the abdominal organs move back, so the horse breathes in. When the horse lands, its head drops, the impact of its forelimbs hitting the ground compresses the chest and the abdominal muscles contract to push the gut forwards, so the horse breathes out.

Chapter 6

The back

Introduction (Fig. 6.1)

The back is that part of the spine between the neck and the tail; it supports the thorax and abdomen suspended beneath it. In the pregnant mare it also supports the weight of her unborn foal. However, it is not designed to carry the weight of a rider and a well-fitting saddle is essential to minimise back problems. The strength of the back results from the combination of bones, ligaments, tendons and muscles, which ensures the spine in this region remains relatively rigid.

The neck (see Chapter 2) and tail are much more flexible than the back. The tail is an active fly swatter and an indicator of discomfort.

Flexibility of the spine (Fig. 6.2)

Contrary to popular belief, the spine from the withers to the top of the tail is only capable of very minor movement in both the up-and-down and side-to-side directions. Such movements can be brought about by the forces transmitted via the hind limbs.

Sometimes movements in one part of the spine are related to movements in another region; for example, when the head and neck are lowered the back appears rounded, whereas when they are raised the back appears hollowed.

Conformation

To be strong the horse's back should be short; a rule of thumb is that there should be no more than a hand's width between the last rib and the point of hip. A horse with a long back will be weak in the loin region and will find it difficult to engage the hindquarters. However, a horse that is very short in the back may lack flexibility.

The entire area of the back is covered by a very dense sheet of deep fascia (a form of connective tissue surrounding muscles and separating groups of muscles). This fascia forms the tendon that attaches to the thoracic and abdominal muscles and attaches to the spinous processes of the thoracic and abdominal processes, merging with the supraspinous ligament. The epaxial muscles lie under this.

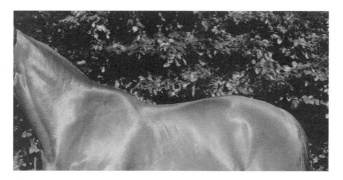

Fig. 6.1   The back – side view

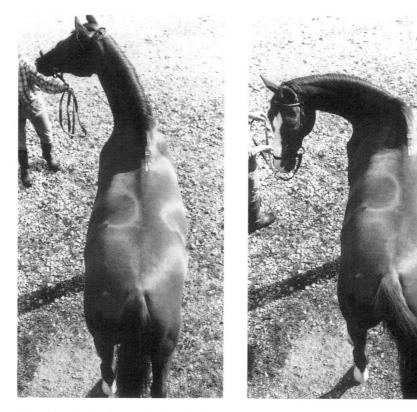

Fig. 6.2   The back is relatively inflexible from withers to tail

The skeleton (Figs 6.3, 6.4)

The vertebral column is the skeleton of the neck, withers, back and tail. Besides support, the main function of the vertebral column is to provide protection for and house the spinal cord, which carries nerve impulses to and from the brain.

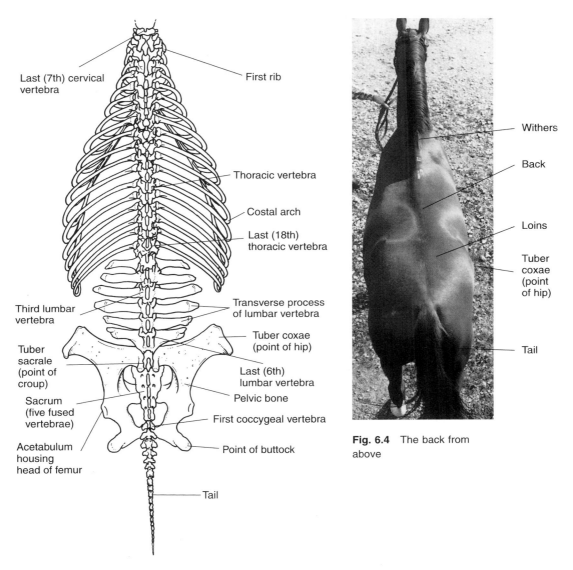

Last (7th) cervical vertebra

First rib

Thoracic vertebra

Costal arch

Last (18th) thoracic vertebra

Third lumbar vertebra

Transverse process of lumbar vertebra

Tuber coxae (point of hip)

Tuber sacrale (point of croup)

Last (6th) lumbar vertebra

Pelvic bone

Sacrum (five fused vertebrae)

First coccygeal vertebra

Acetabulum housing head of femur

Point of buttock

Tail

Fig. 6.3   Vertebral column

Withers

Back

Loins

Tuber coxae (point of hip)

Tail

Fig. 6.4   The back from above

Regions of the spine

The vertebral column can be divided into five regions

- The neck – 7 cervical vertebrae
- Upper back – 18 thoracic vertebrae
- Loins – 6 lumbar vertebrae
- Croup – 5 fused sacral vertebrae
- Tail – 15–20 coccygeal vertebrae.

Vertebrae

The vertebrae make up a long bony chain to protect the spinal cord. At each vertebra a pair of spinal nerves branches off from the spinal cord to penetrate every part of the horse's body. Muscles are attached by their ligaments to the lateral and articular processes of the vertebrae so enabling the horse to move. The spinal cord ends in the middle of the sacrum where it sends out nerves to supply the horse's tail.

Structure of the vertebrae

Each vertebra has the same basic shape:

*   The vertebral main body or centrum
*   An arch surmounted by the dorsal spine
*   A pair of transverse processes of variable size and shape
*   Two pairs of articular surfaces.

Intervertebral discs

The degree of movement of the spine depends on the thickness of the intervertebral discs that are firmly attached between the vertebrae. As the horse gets older the discs become calcified, thus joining the vertebrae together. There may even be further outgrowths of bone acting as bridges across neighbouring vertebrae.

Cervical vertebrae

The cervical vertebrae were described in Chapter 2.

Thoracic vertebrae (Fig. 6.5)

There are 18 thoracic vertebrae, each separated by cartilaginous interverte-bral discs. The spinous processes are very large, giving the horse its pro-nounced withers and allowing extensive muscle and ligament attachment.

The withers: The withers are the highest point of the thoracic spine and are formed by the third to the tenth thoracic vertebrae. The withers are held firmly in place by ligaments between the vertebral spines and other muscles and ligaments attached to them, including part of the nuchal ligament.

Movement between the horse's thoracic vertebrae is strictly limited.

Lumbar vertebrae (Fig. 6.6)

The lumbar vertebrae make up the loins region. There are normally six lumbar vertebrae but sometimes only five; in same breeds, particularly the Arab, an extra thoracic vertebra is often found.

The width of the transverse processes and the length of the dorsal spines characterise the lumbar vertebrae. The lumbar vertebrae of the

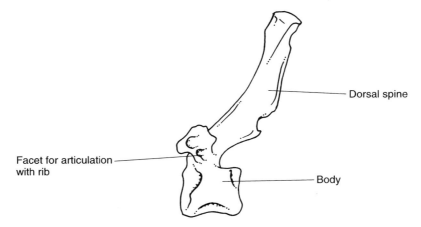

Dorsal spine

Facet for articulation
with rib

Body

Fig. 6.5 Thoracic vertebra – side view

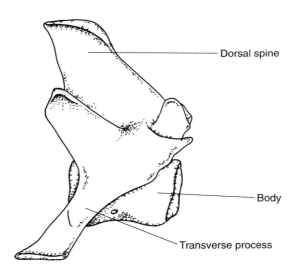

Dorsal spine

Body

Transverse process

Fig. 6.6 Lumbar vertebra – side view

horse carry three extra articular facets, making the horse different from most other mammals; these limit movement of the spine in the lumbar region. However, it should be remembered that:

- The loins are the most flexible and vulnerable part of the back.
- A well-designed and correctly fitting saddle, ensuring the rider's weight is not taken on the loins or the vertebral column, will help to protect the horse's back.

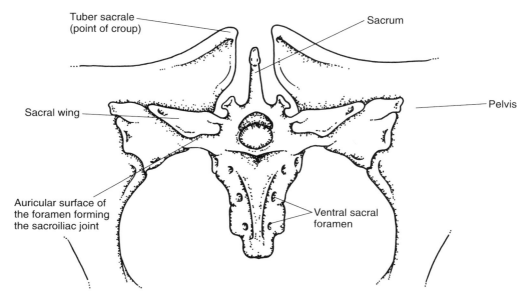

Fig. 6.7   Sacrum – view through the pelvis

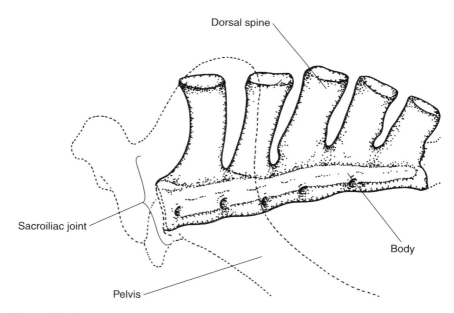

Fig. 6.8   Sacral vertebra – side view

Sacrum (Figs 6.7, 6.8)

The triangular sacrum is a composite bone made up of five vertebrae which fuse together when the horse is 4 or 5 years old. The sacrum forms an integral part of the pelvic girdle, providing a firm link between the hindquarters and the trunk. The first sacral vertebra has an enlarged transverse process called the sacral wing which forms a synovial joint, the lumbosacral joint, with the transverse process of the 6th lumbar vertebra; the underside of the sacral wing forms the sacroiliac joint with the ilium of the pelvic bone.

Coccygeal vertebrae (Fig. 6.9)

There are normally 18 coccygeal or tail vertebrae, but the number can vary from 15 to 21. They decrease in size from the first to the last.

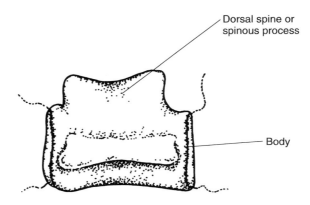

Dorsal spine or spinous process

Body

Fig. 6.9 Coccygeal vertebra – side view

Joints

Sacroiliac joint (Fig. 6.10)

This joint is a combined synovial and fibrocartilaginous joint and does not move. It is supported by ventral, dorsal and lateral sacroiliac ligaments.

Lumbosacral joint

The lumbosacral joint is part of the spine and acts to transmit the impulsion generated by the hindquarters. Its flexibility, although limited, allows the pelvis to rotate forwards under the horse's body during canter and gallop and when engaging the hindquarters to raise the back. This rotation mainly takes place when both hind limbs move forwards. Even though the lumbosacral joint has limited action, the ability of the horse to move well is dependent upon its full function.

At the walk and trot both hind legs move in opposite directions; because the lumbosacral joint is incapable of sideways flexion some of this movement is taken up by the sacroiliac joints. For maximum effectiveness

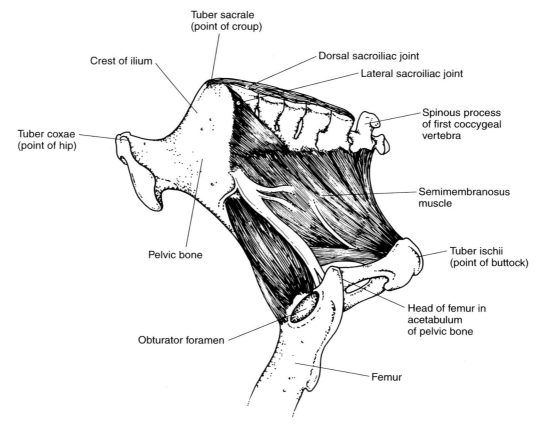

Fig. 6.10 Sacroiliac joint – side view

the lumbosacral joint should be positioned as far as possible in front of the sacroiliac prominences (point of croup). If a horse's back is long, there is additional leverage on the lumbosacral joint, increasing the stress put on the area by the rider's weight and the demands of engagement. This area can be supported and strengthened with the correct muscle development.

Ligaments

The ligaments of the spine are important in helping to keep the individual vertebrae in place and giving the back strength and stability.

Supraspinous ligament

The supraspinous ligament runs along the back from the sacrum and joins together the top of the spinous processes of all of the lumbar and thoracic vertebrae. In the withers area the ligaments flatten to form a broad sheet, extending on either side almost to the scapular cartilages.

Nuchal ligament

In the neck the supraspinous ligament is modified to form the nuchal ligament, which is strong and elastic. The lamellar part of the nuchal ligament is made up of two sheets running down either side of the neck which attach to the cervical vertebrae. The funicular part runs from the withers up the neck to the poll where it attaches to the occiput of the skull. Where the ligament runs over the withers the supraspinous bursa, which contains lubricating synovial fluid, reduces friction; this lies between the second and fourth thoracic spinous processes and is the site associated with the condition termed fistulous withers.

Sacroiliac ligaments

These support the sacroiliac joint.

Musculature

Trapezius

The trapezius is a flattended triangular sheet of superfircial muscle, the base of which arises in the area of the neck, withers and thorax from the funicular part of the nuchal ligament and the supraspinous ligament, back to the tenth thoracic vertebra. The thoracic part of the trapezius muscle originates on the thoracic vertebrae and inserts onto the scapula. As stated in Chapter 3, its action is to draw the scapula up and back to lift the shoulder.

Latissimus dorsi

The latissimus dorsi lies behind the shoulder covering the side of the chest and extending up onto the back. The muscle passes from the upper part of the thorax onto the rear of the humerus and its action is to pull the forelimb back (see Chapter 3). When the forefoot is on the ground, contraction of the latissimus dorsi moves the body forwards over the limb.

Both the trapezius and latissimus dorsi are large flat sheets of muscle; the fibres tend to be long and run more or less parallel to the long axis and their attaching tendons are also sheet-like. Because the range of movement of a muscle depends on the length of its constituent fibres, sheet muscles like these produce large movements.

Epaxials

The epaxial muscle mass helps convert the backbone from a chain of individual bones to a rigid structure, strong enough to carry the gut and to transmit the power from the hindquarters to the front end of the horse. The epaxial muscles are made up of three main components: the iliocostal and longissimus in the back and loins; the spinal and semispinal parts of the transversospinal component in the back and neck.

Longissimus dorsi (thoracic, lumbar regions)

The longissimus dorsi is the largest and longest muscle in the horse's body. It helps to form the contours of the horse's back, running from the pelvis and sacrum along the back to insert on the thoracic vertebrae. This is the muscle on which the saddle, and hence the rider, sits. Its role is to transmit to the forehand the propulsion generated by the hind limbs.

The epaxial and logissimus dorsi muscles control the movement of the back. Thus the flexor (abdominal) muscles contract to extend the back (round) and the extensor muscles (muscles along the top of the spine) contract to flex (hollow) it. These movements are minor.

Nerves

The spinal nerves make up a regular series of 42 pairs that arise from the spinal cord. There are

- 18 pairs of thoracic spinal nerves
- 6 pairs of lumbar spinal nerves.

The spinal nerves carry messages from the spinal cord to the muscles and skin of the limbs and from there back to the spinal cord.

Back injuries and their prevention

The horse is designed to move forward at high speed, rather than to jump and move laterally as is required in dressage. The muscles of the back are therefore particularly prone to injury when the horse is asked to carry out difficult manoeuvres.

When working a horse the aim is to round and strengthen the back and engage the hindquarters. A horse's back becomes slightly rounded when the abdominal and spinal flexor muscles are used. The contraction of the abdominal muscles tilts the horse's pelvis and brings the hindquarters more underneath the abdomen. To tilt the pelvis there must be some movement in the lumbosacral and sacroiliac areas together with movement of the associated ligaments. Injury of the sacroiliac ligaments is a common cause of back pain in horses. The 'jumper's bump', where the point of the croup (sacral tuber of the ilium) becomes overly prominent may be a sign of long-term sacroiliac problems.

As with most sports injuries the problem can be avoided by:

- Thorough warm-up
- Increasing the difficulty of exercises gradually
- Giving short periods of walking and stretching during schooling
- Avoiding tension
- Avoiding fatigue
- Cooling down thoroughly.

Part 2

The Horse in Action

Chapter 7

Movement and action

Biomechanics

Biomechanics is the study of movement, knowledge of which enables the rider or trainer to make an objective assessment of the way the horse moves. This, combined with a good knowledge of anatomy and conformation, allows the training programme to be designed to prolong the horse's working life. The first thing to do is to identify the weak or problem areas and then work the horse in such a way as to strengthen these areas. In this way the horse will be able to realise its potential without over-stress and is more likely to stay mentally and physically sound.

Anatomical points affecting movement and action

The following points all affect the way the horse moves:

- The front legs are attached to the rib-cage by muscles and ligaments, not by a collar bone. Instead the horse's body is slung in a cradle of muscle between the two shoulder blades. These muscles allow the horse's trunk to rise and fall or to lean a little to one side, helping the horse keep its balance, particularly when cornering at speed.
- The front legs bear more weight than the hind legs, and hence there is more concussion involved with the movement.
- The head and neck act as a balancing weight.
- The muscles which bring the front legs forward are attached to the neck.
- The spine has limited sideways and up and down movement between the neck and tail. In practical terms the trunk is almost rigid, and its role is to transfer the power generated by the hind legs into forward motion.
- The hind legs have a bony attachment to the spine for effective transfer of the forces of movement.

Gaits

Each gait has a characteristic sequence of footfalls, which determines the number of beats per stride and gives rise to the rhythm of the gait.

- Tempo is used to describe either the speed of the rhythm or the velocity of the gait.
- Cadence is used to indicate that a gait combines rhythm with impulsion.

Gaits can be described as symmetric or asymmetric. In a symmetric gait right and left sides move in a similar way.

The gait cycle

During locomotion the horse's limbs undergo repeated cycles of movement called strides. The stride length is measured from placement to placement of the same foot. The stride can be divided into different phases; for example, the stance phase occurs when the limb is in contact with the ground, and the swing phase when the limb is being carried through the air.

Swing phase
In the swing phase the limb is pulled forwards and then backwards before initial ground contact. The purpose of this 'swing phase retraction' is to reduce the speed of the hoof at initial ground contact. During the swing phase the limbs act like pendulums. The forelimb rotates with its pivot point in the upper part of the scapula. The hind limb rotates around the hip joint in the walk and trot, and around the lumbosacral joint (just in front of the croup) in the canter and gallop. Moving the point of rotation from the hip joint to the lumbosacral joint increases the effective length of the hind limbs and therefore increases the stride length.

Stance phase
The stance phase is the period during which the hoof is in contact with the ground. Each limb has a stance phase in every stride. The stance phase consists of:

- Initial ground contact
- Impact phase
- Loading phase
- Breakover.

Initial ground contact: the initial contact may be heel first or flat footed in the slow gaits, whereas in racing gaits the heel usually contacts the ground first. In some movements, such as piaffe, toe first contacts are normal.

Impact phase: the impact phase occupies the first few milliseconds after the hoof contacts the ground. During this time the limb undergoes rapid deceleration, causing a shock wave to travel up the horse's limb. The impact phase is so short that the muscles do not have sufficient time to respond and protect the bones and joints.

Loading phase: after the foot has contacted the ground, the horse's body weight passes over the limb. From the time the hoof contacts the ground to mid-stance when the horse's body weight is positioned directly over the limb, there is a deceleration or breaking phase. During this time the deep and superficial digital flexor tendons and the suspensory ligament are stretched. Mid-stance occurs when the cannon bone is vertical and the fetlock sinks to its lowest point. After mid-stance the tension in the flexor tendons and the suspensory ligament is reduced, and they start to recoil elastically, helping to flex the lower limbs during the swing phase.

Breakover: this begins when the heels leave the ground and start to rotate around the toe of the hoof, which is still in contact with the ground. On a hard surface, the hoof remains flat on the ground until the heel is off. On a softer surface the toe rotates into the surface before heel-off which reduces pressure in the navicular region. Toe-off is the instant at which the toe leaves the ground, after which the elastic tendons and ligaments are able to recoil in an unrestrained manner. As the toe pushes off there is an acceleration or propulsive phase from mid-stance to take-off.

Chapter 8

Walking

Footfall sequence of the walk

This chapter examines the slowest of the horse's gaits, the walk. Each gait has a characteristic sequence of footfalls and movements (Fig. 8.1). The walk consists of eight different movements. The horse in turn stands on the:

- Left hind, left fore, right hind (hind triple stance)
- Two diagonal legs – right hind, left fore (right diagonal double stance)
- Left fore, right hind, right fore (fore triple stance)
- Two right lateral legs – right hind, right fore (right lateral double stance)
- Left hind, right hind, right fore (hind triple stance)
- Two diagonal legs – left hind, right fore (left diagonal double stance)
- Right fore, left hind, left fore (fore triple stance)
- Two left lateral legs – left hind, left fore (left lateral double stance).

The rider is aware of this as a four-time beat which should have a regular and even rhythm.

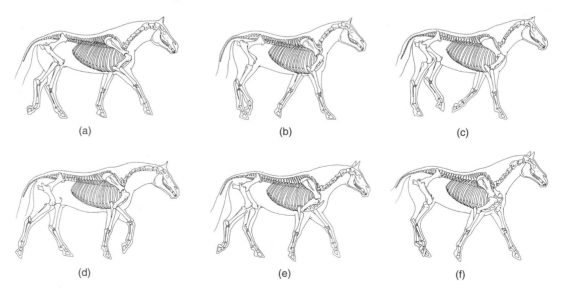

(a)   (b)   (c)

(d)   (e)   (f)

Fig. 8.1 Footfall sequence of the walk

Walking on the right rein

Hind triple stance

In the series of illustrations shown here, the horse starts the walk on the right rein, with the horse placing the right hind leg on the ground. The horse is now standing on three limbs, the right and left hind and the left fore (Fig. 8.2).

Right diagonal double stance

The left hind leg is then lifted, leaving the horse standing on two limbs: the right hind and the left fore (Fig. 8.3).

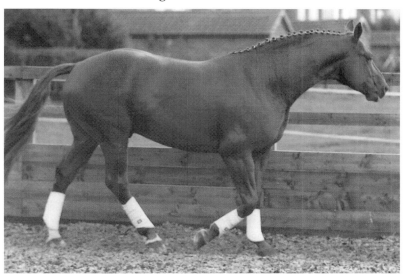

Fig. 8.2 Right hind impact

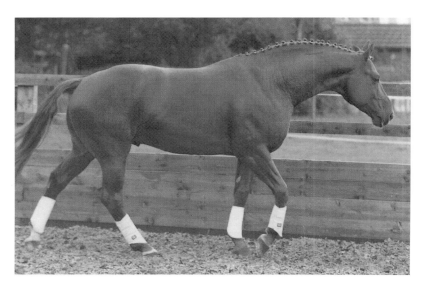

Fig. 8.3 Left hind lift-off

Fore triple stance

The right foreleg is then set down, so that the horse is again standing on three legs: the right fore, left fore and right hind (Fig. 8.4).

Fig. 8.5 shows the skeletal system and Fig. 8.6 shows the musculature of the same horse at the same point in the walk stride as Fig. 8.4. The bones involved are illustrated in Fig. 1.3.

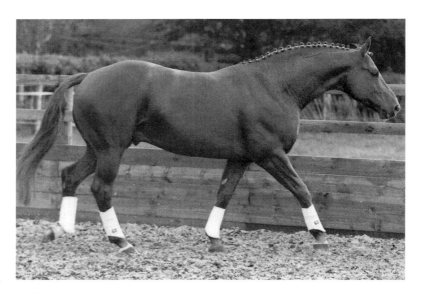

Fig. 8.4   Right fore impact

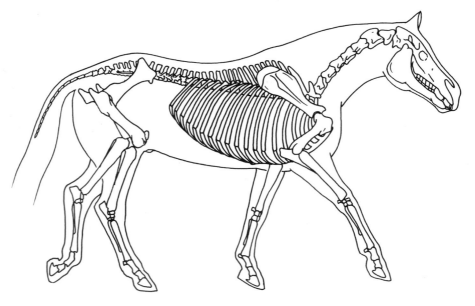

Fig. 8.5   Right fore impact – skeleton

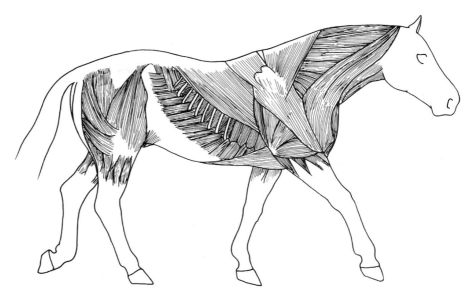

Fig. 8.6 Right fore impact – musculature

Right lateral double stance

In Fig. 8.7 the left fore is lifted off the ground, leaving the horse standing on the right hind and right fore limbs, a position known as the *right lateral double stance*. Figs 8.8 and 8.9 show the skeleton and musculature, respectively, involved in the left fore lift-off. Fig. 8.10 shows the position of the right lateral double stance while Fig. 8.11 shows the skeleton and Fig. 8.12 shows the musculature.

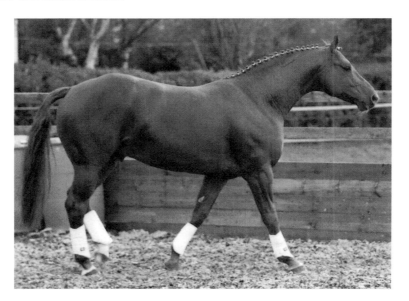

Fig. 8.7 Left fore lift-off

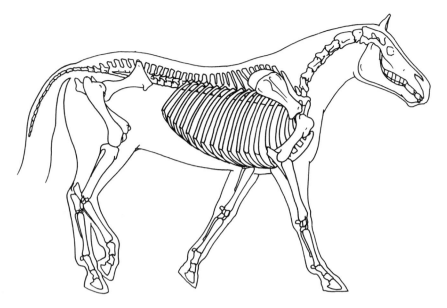

Fig. 8.8   Left fore lift-off – skeleton

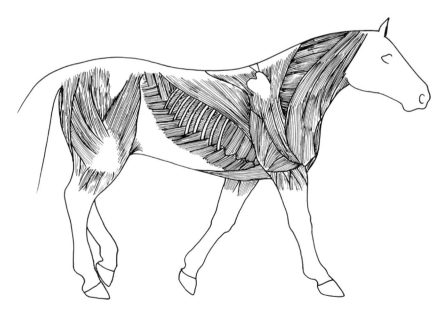

Fig. 8.9   Left fore lift-off – musculature

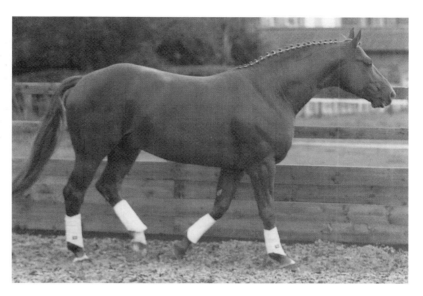

Fig. 8.10 Right lateral double stance

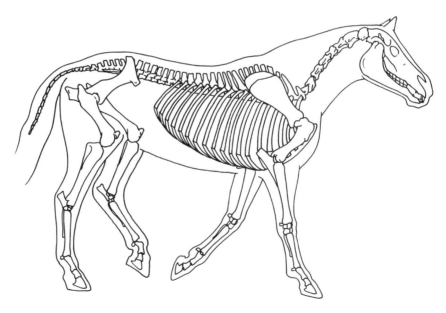

Fig. 8.11 Right lateral double stance – skeleton

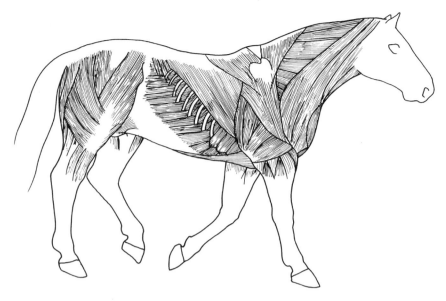

Fig. 8.12 Right lateral double stance – musculature

Left diagonal double stance

The left hind leg then hits the ground so that the horse is again standing on three legs: both hind legs and the right fore. This is the *hind triple stance* again, but with different limbs involved compared with the first hind triple stance. Following this, the right hind lifts off. In Fig. 8.13 the right hind is lifted off the ground to leave the left hind and the right fore on the ground. Figs 8.14 and 8.15 show the skeleton and musculature involved in the right hind lift-off, while Figs 8.16–8.18 show the left diagonal double stance itself.

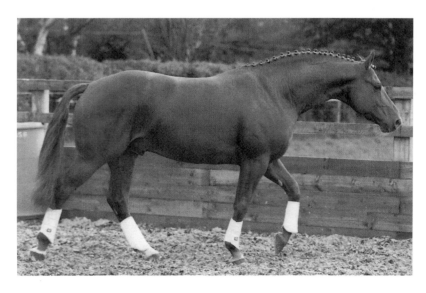

Fig. 8.13 Right hind lift-off

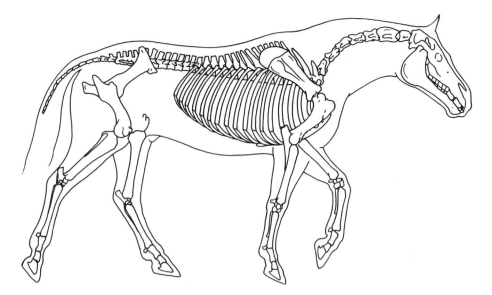

Fig. 8.14   Right hind lift-off – skeleton

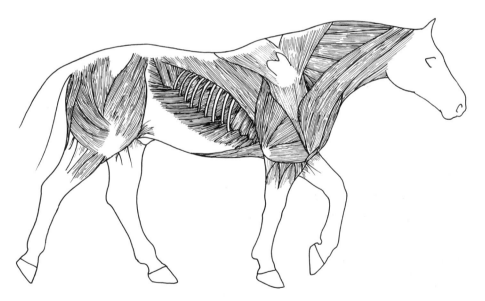

Fig. 8.15   Right hind lift-off – musculature

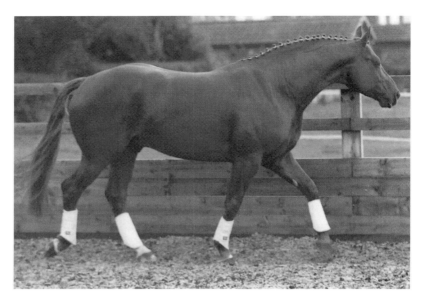

Fig. 8.16   Left diagonal double stance

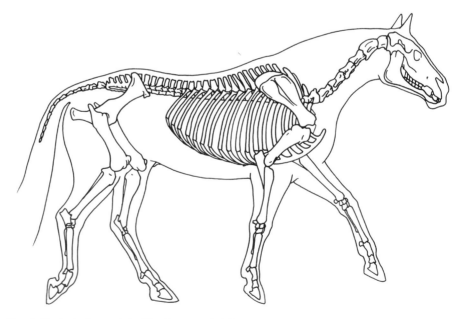

Fig. 8.17   Left diagonal double stance – skeleton

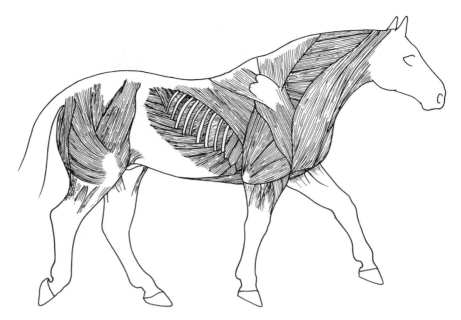

Fig. 8.18 Left diagonal double stance – musculature

Fore triple stance

The left diagonal double stance is followed by the left foreleg hitting the ground, so that the horse is again standing on three legs: right fore, left hind and right fore. Note that this fore triple stance uses a different combination of limbs from that earlier in the sequence.

Left lateral double stance

Our sequence is concluded in Fig. 8.19, which shows the right fore about to be lifted off the ground. This is the start of the left lateral double stance, which leaves the horse standing on the left hind and left fore. Figs 8.20 and 8.21 show the skeleton and musculature involved in the lift-off.

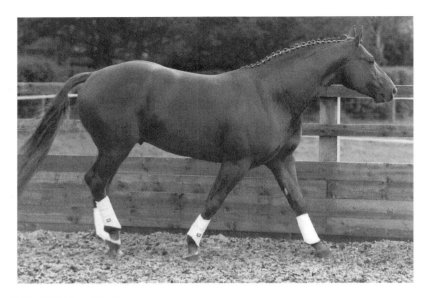

Fig. 8.19   Right fore lift-off

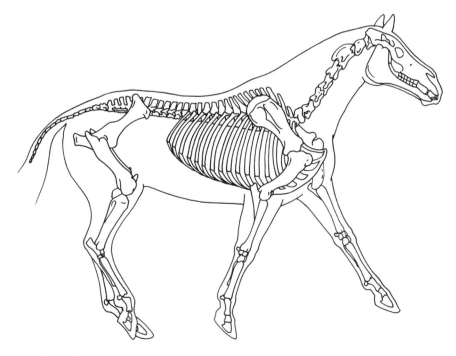

Fig. 8.20   Right fore lift-off – skeleton

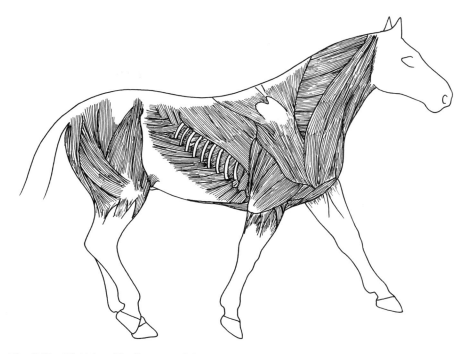

Fig. 8.21 Right fore lift-off – musculature

Moving the forelimb forwards

The front leg is moved forwards by two main groups of muscles which bend the elbows forwards and pull the leg forwards. The elbow is flexed by the:

- Biceps – running from the scapula to the radius
- Brachialis – running from the humerus to the radius.

The forelimb is pulled forwards by the combined action of the:

- Brachiocephalicus muscle – running from the atlas vertebra to the humerus, which pulls the humerus forwards
- Serratus ventralis (thoracic) muscle – running from the scapula to the ribs, which pulls the scapula down and backwards.

All these muscles are illustrated in Figs 5.4 and 5.5.

Lifting the foot

Flexors at the back of the knee contract to flex the knee and digital joints and, as the knee moves forwards and upwards, the foot is lifted from the ground. The leg is now suspended from the withers by the dorsal scapular ligaments and the trapezius muscle.

Knee action

As the leg is lifted, it folds. Heavy shoes or long toes will increase the amount of folding. Thus, hackneys are shod with heavy shoes to increase their knee action, while racehorses are shod with light aluminium plates to minimise knee action.

Straightening the forelimb

After the limb has moved forward sufficiently it is straightened again.

- The shoulder is straightened by the supraspinatus muscle which runs from the scapula to the humerus
- The elbow is straightened by the triceps
- The lower leg (knee, fetlock, pastern and coffin joints) is straightened by the carpal and digital extensor muscles.

The limb is rigid as it hits the ground. The foot acts as a pivot over which the body can move so that the impetus of the body above the foot drives the horse forwards.

Moving the hind limb forwards

Movement of the hind limb differs from that of the forelimb because there is a direct connection from the pelvis to the vertebral column. Initially the hind limb is brought forwards by flexion of the hip joint (Fig. 8.6), which in turn carries the femur and stifle forwards; during this movement the stifle is also flexed, which in turn flexes the hock. The gluteal muscles which give the hindquarters their rounded shape and the biceps femoris which lies below them, extend the hip joint. The semitendinosus flexes the stifle, while the hock is flexed through the action of the peroneus tertius muscle. Contraction of the tibialis anterior muscles also contributes to hock and stifle flexion.

After the limb has moved forwards sufficiently (Fig. 8.9), the stifle is extended by the quadriceps femoris group of muscles (Fig. 8.12). At the same time, the hock extends through the reciprocal mechanism of the tendinous superficial flexor and the tendinous cord in the gastrocnemius muscle.

Straightening the hind limb

When the foot hits the ground (Fig. 8.15) the hind limb is locked into position; muscles pull the rigid limb backwards and strongly stabilise the stifle and hip joints (Fig. 8.18). The limb is turned on the head of the femur, extending the hip joint (Figs 8.12 and 8.21). As the limb approaches the vertical, the stifle and hock flex slightly and the fetlock sinks to aid shock absorption.

When the limb passes the vertical, the rump and hamstring (semi-tendinosus, semimembranosus and biceps femoris) muscles extend the hip, stifle and hock. The semitendinosus lies to the rear of the gluteal muscles, separated by a groove known as the poverty line because it becomes distinct in lean horses.

As soon as the hoof leaves the ground, elastic rebound of the peroneus tertius and tibialis anterior system returns the hock to semiflexion so that the limb is ready to be brought forwards again.

Qualities of a good walk

The quality and regularity of the walk should be judged throughout the eight movements.

- There is a regular, four-time beat
- Each foot is placed firmly and squarely on the ground without hesitation and with plenty of impulsion
- The interval between the leg being raised and lowered should be the same for each leg
- Strides should be even, purposeful and not constrained
- The legs are lifted, not dragged along the ground
- The head should be free to move and not constrained by the rider.

Impulsion

Too little impulsion results in the horse dragging his toes, particularly the hind toes. Too much uncontrolled impulsion can result in the horse rushing as the feet hurry to keep up with each other. This often leads to unevenly sized steps and a loss of rhythm. Sometimes, horses will develop a two-time walk with the limbs moving as lateral pairs. This is a major fault and can be difficult to correct.

The benefits of walking

The horse uses a vast number of muscles when walking without putting them under stress; the muscles contract and relax regularly, encouraging good circulation. In an active walk the horse's back pulsates and swings, helping to remove tension and muscle bunching, making it ideal relaxation between bouts of more strenuous exercise.

The walk in dressage

The walk in dressage terms has four variations:

- Free
- Extended
- Medium
- Collected.

In the medium walk the horse travels at 100–110 m/min, taking strides about 1.65 m in length.

Collection

The sequence of steps stays the same in the free, extended, medium and collected walks. However, in collected walk the horse should move with a short and cadenced step and the pace should be regular and even. It is not uncommon for the horse to lose this regularity as more collection is demanded.

Over tracking

Horses with long limbs and a short-coupled body tend to show a marked degree of over tracking, where the hind foot contacts the ground in front of the forefoot on the same side (ipsilateral). Consequently, as the stride length increases, the forefoot must be raised relatively early in the stride to avoid interference by the hind foot.

Over reaching

At walk there is plenty of time for the left forelimb to get out of the way before the left hind limb hits the ground. As the speed of the gait increases there is less time for this to happen so that the limbs are more likely to interfere, leading to *forging* or *over reaching*. Forging occurs when the hind shoe strikes the toe of the front shoe, with a characteristic noise.

The walk with rider

Fig. 8.22 shows right foreleg about to be set down, so that the horse is changing from right diagonal double stance with two feet on the ground to fore triple stance with three feet on the ground. The position of the horse is equivalent to that shown in Fig. 8.4. The rider is allowing the horse to walk forwards freely on a loose rein contact. Although the horse has brought his nose back to the vertical and shortened his neck slightly, the stride length remains the same as that of the unridden horse in Fig. 8.4.

Figures 8.23 and 8.24 show the underlying structures of muscle and bone. The saddle is placed over the thoracic vertebrae. The spinous processes of the thoracic vertebrae of horses with high withers are pronounced, increasing the chance of the saddle putting pressure on this area. The horse in Fig. 8.22 has a large shoulder with the scapula showing a slope of about 45°, so there may be a problem here with finding a saddle that does not interfere with the free movement of the shoulder. However, in Fig. 8.22 it is clear that this dressage saddle sits behind the horse's scapula and does not restrict his movement in any way. The area of back behind the saddle consists of the thoracic vertebrae and ribs do not support these. A saddle that sits too far back will rest on this weaker area. In a horse such as the one in Fig. 8.22, with a relatively short back and a good shoulder, there is little room to fit a saddle correctly.

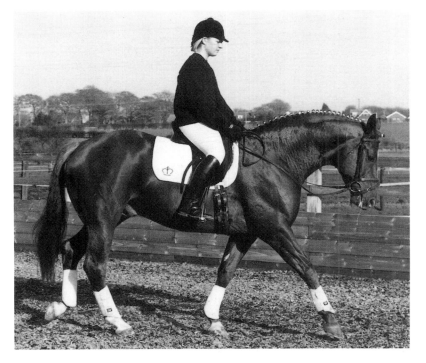

Fig. 8.22   Right fore impact of horse with rider

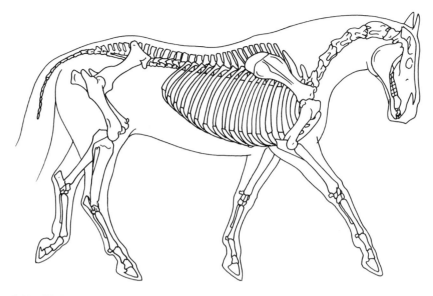

Fig. 8.23 Right fore impact of ridden horse – skeleton

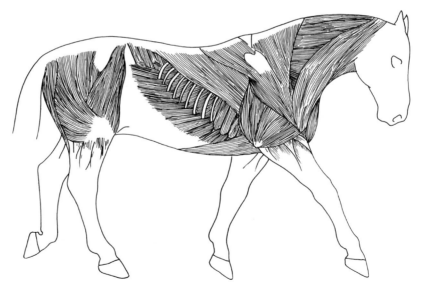

Fig. 8.24 Right fore impact of ridden horse – musculature

Chapter 9

Trotting

Characteristics of the trot

- Medium speed gait.
- Two-time beat.
- Legs move in diagonal pairs with a period of suspension when all the limbs are off the ground. The period of suspension is the part when the rider is usually rising out of the saddle.
- Symmetrical gait.

Closer examination of the trot shows that the left and right sides move as mirror images, the diagonal limbs move more or less synchronously and there are usually two airborne phases per stride.

Qualities of a good trot

- Regular two-time beat
- Strides even in length and not hurried
- Hindquarters engaged
- The hind feet do not hit the forefeet (forging)
- Light, elastic and balanced
- Knees and hocks flex freely and at the same height
- The horse should not drag its toes
- The rhythm should be the same on a straight line and on a circle
- The head should remain steady
- The fore and hind limbs should be equally active.

A good trot depends on a supple back, good balance, engagement of the hindquarters and elastic, supple joints. The trot is not correct if the two support legs do not hit the ground at the same time. For example, the hind limb may touch down before the forelimb.

Footfall sequence of the trot

The characteristic footfall sequence of the trot is, left hind with right fore, and right hind with left fore (Fig. 9.1).

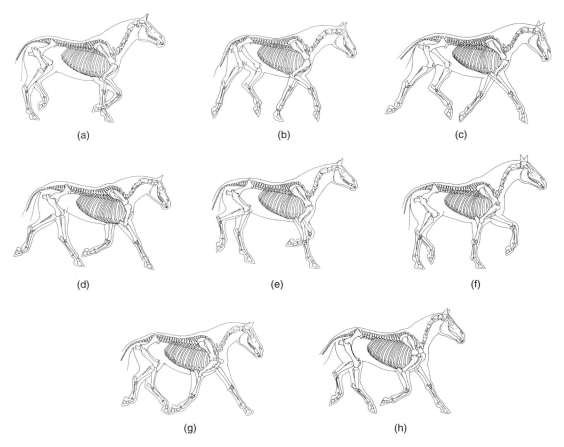

(a)   (b)   (c)

(d)   (e)   (f)

(g)   (h)

Fig. 9.1 Footfall sequence of the trot

Right diagonal stance

In Fig. 9.2 (p. 101) the left fore and right hind are in contact with the ground. This is known as the *right diagonal stance*. The diagonal is named from the hind foot on the ground. Figs 9.3 and 9.4 show the skeleton and musculature at this point in the sequence.

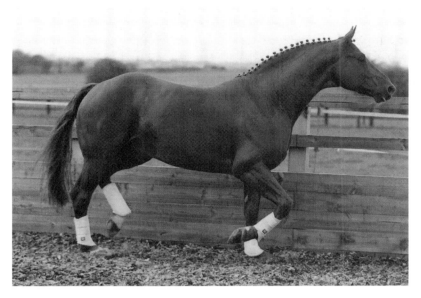

Fig. 9.2   Right diagonal double stance

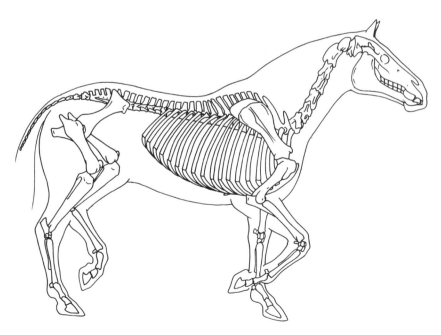

Fig. 9.3   Right diagonal double stance – skeleton

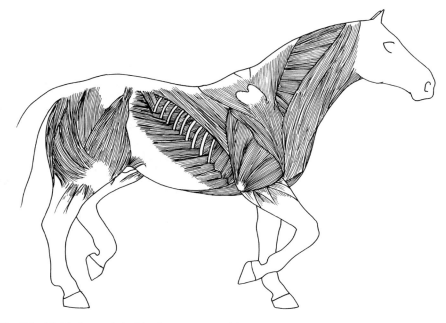

Fig. 9.4 Right diagonal double stance – musculature

Left fore single stance

In Fig. 9.5 (p. 103) the right hind foot has left the ground momentarily before the left fore, which is still in contact with the ground. This is the *left fore single stance*. Figures 9.6 and 9.7 show the skeleton and musculature at the point of right hind lift-off.

Raising the forehand

To raise a forelimb it helps if the centre of gravity is first moved back. In this way, the horse raises its head and neck and contraction of the serratus ventralis raises the thorax on the side on which the muscles are acting. This places extra weight onto that foreleg and relieves the opposite foreleg of enough weight to permit the elbow to flex and the joint to be moved forwards. At the same time, contraction of the anterior deep pectoral muscles between the front legs also raises the thorax. Flexion in the hocks, which may be almost imperceptible, occurs and the resulting drop of even a few centimetres in the hindquarters is sufficient to move the centre of gravity back and release significant weight from the forehand.

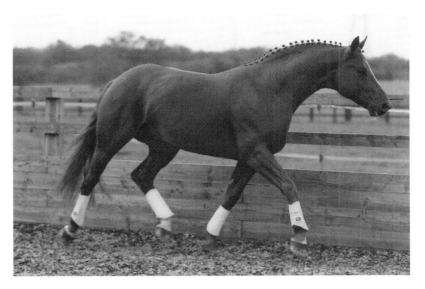

Fig. 9.5   Right hind lift-off

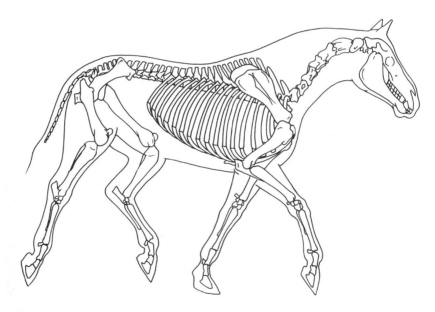

Fig. 9.6   Right hind lift-off – skeleton

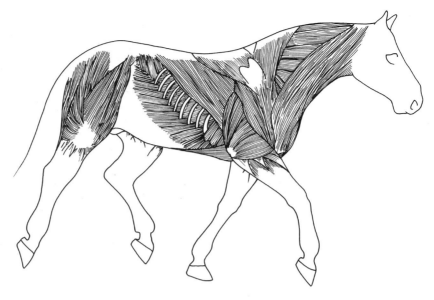

Fig. 9.7   Right hind lift-off – musculature

First suspension phase

In Figs 9.8–9.10 (pp. 105–6) the left fore is lifting off the ground just before the first suspension or airborne phase during which the horse is able to cover the ground. Young horses sometimes show less suspension than trained animals. This young horse has natural impulsion and rhythm and clearly demonstrates the suspension phase. The suspension should not lift the horse up without taking it forwards.

Forearm extensor muscles

The muscles that extend the foreleg can be clearly seen in Fig. 9.8. They are the:

- Radial carpal extensor muscle at the front of the leg
- Common digital extensor muscle behind it.

Digital extensor tendon

Only the tendons from the forearm muscles extend down below the knee. In Fig. 9.8 the common digital extensor tendon can be seen at the base of the common digital extensor muscle. This tendon runs down over the knee, joins the lateral digital extensor tendon and attaches to the pedal bone in the foot.

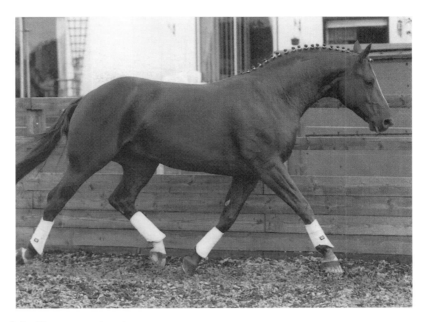

Fig. 9.8   First suspension phase

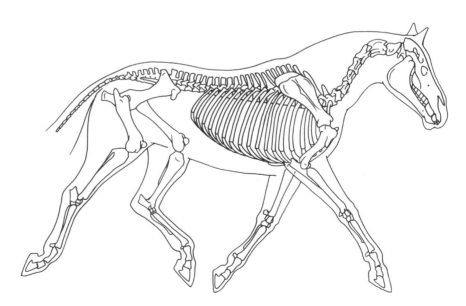

Fig. 9.9   First suspension phase – skeleton

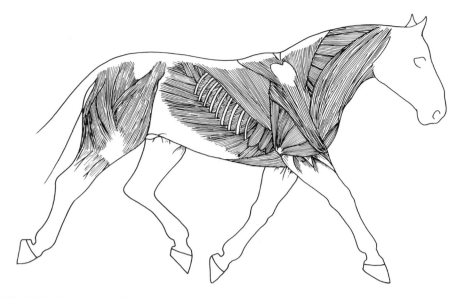

Fig. 9.10 First suspension phase – musculature

End of first suspension phase

In Figs 9.11 and 9.12 (p. 107) the left fore has lifted off and all four feet are off the ground and the left hind is preparing to make contact. Figure 9.13 shows the left hind limb making contact with the ground slightly before the right fore lands, so that the horse's weight is taken on one limb momentarily. This is *left hind single stance*. The fetlock is extended so that the digits are in a straight line with the leg when the foot lands (Fig. 9.14).

Collection and suspension
As the trot becomes more collected there must be sufficient impulsion to maintain the suspension so that the freedom of the trot is not lost. The sequence remains unchanged in the variations of the trot but the length of stride and duration of the suspension alter. A slow trot or jog has little or no suspension, while in the dressage horse the suspension should be obvious.

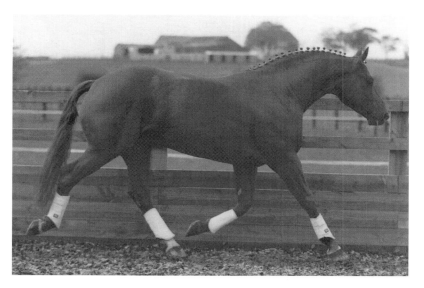

Fig. 9.11   End of first suspension phase

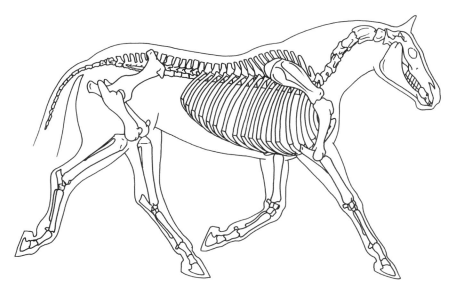

Fig. 9.12   End of first suspension phase – skeleton

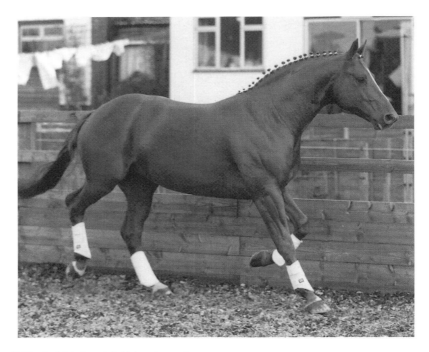

Fig. 9.13 Left hind and right fore impact

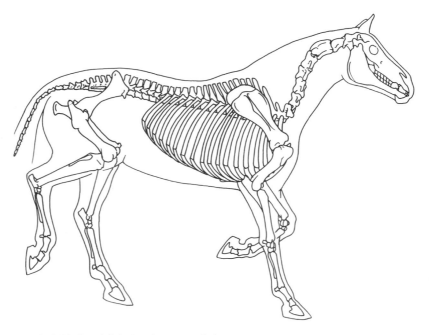

Fig. 9.14 Left hind and right fore impact – skeleton

Left diagonal double stance

In Fig. 9.15 the right fore has made contact and the horse has the left diagonal feet on the ground. This is followed by lift-off of the left hind, leaving the right fore the only foot on the ground for a short period of time. Fig. 9.16 shows the skeleton at this point in the sequence.

Shock absorption

When the foot is on the ground the fetlock sinks, as shown in Fig. 9.15. The suspensory ligament, then the superficial flexor tendon, then the deep flexor tendon and finally the check ligament control this movement. These tendons and ligaments help to reduce shock (by absorbing the energy of the impact) and to add smoothness to the action. The fetlock recovers when the leg has passed over the vertical. In this way the limb is shortened and lengthened, helping to keep the body at nearly the same level throughout the stride.

Propulsion

As the horse's leg leaves the ground, deep flexor muscles pull the pedal bone back with such energy that the rotation of the coffin joint and the upward movement of the fetlock add forward propulsive force to the stride. This is assisted by the elasticity of the suspensory ligament.

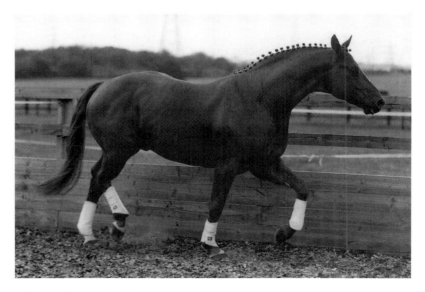

Fig. 9.15 Left diagonal double stance

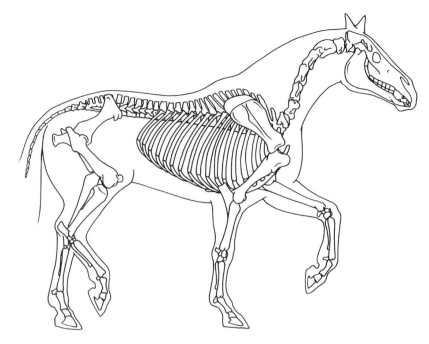

Fig. 9.16 Left diagonal double stance – skeleton

Second suspension phase

In Fig. 9.17 the right fore has lifted off the ground and the horse is in the second suspension phase of the stride. The way in which the horse extends the left fore and right hind to produce the longer stride needed for an extended trot is clearly demonstrated. Figs 9.18 and 9.19 show the skeleton and musculature at this point in the sequence.

The hamstring muscles
The extensors or hamstring group of muscles of the hindquarters include:

- Biceps femoris – the most important of the hamstring muscles, running from the sacral vertebrae to the femur
- Semitendinosus – running from the pelvis to the tibia
- Semimembranosus – running from the pelvis to the femur.

The deep medial gluteal muscle, running from the top of the pelvis to the femur, is also a strong hip extensor.

Hip joint flexors include:

- Superficial gluteal muscle
- Quadriceps femoris – made up of four parts
- Tensor fascia latae.

The gluteal muscles and the biceps femoris extend the femur as the hind leg pushes off from the ground. The gluteal muscles also flex the stifle joint, which in turn causes hock flexion.

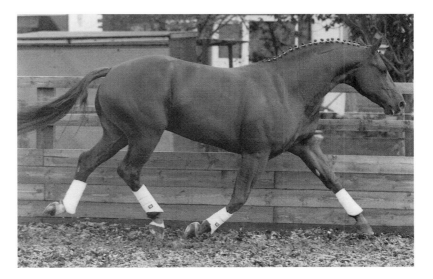

Fig. 9.17   Second suspension phase

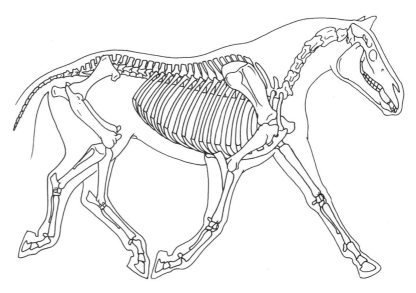

Fig. 9.18   Second suspension phase – skeleton

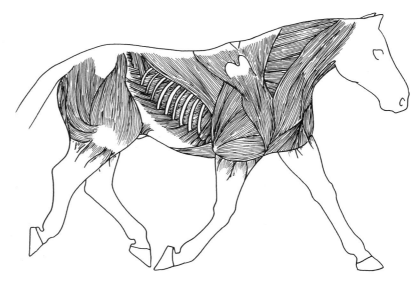

Fig. 9.19 Second suspension phase – musculature

End of the second suspension phase

The moment just before the right hind hits the ground is shown in Fig. 9.20 and Fig. 9.21. The left fore hitting the ground and the start of the subsequent stride will follow this.

Hind lower limb extension

The muscles that extend the lower leg forwards make up the horse's second thigh (Fig. 9.20) are the:

- Long digital extensor muscle at the front
- Lateral digital extensor muscle behind it.

They attach to the extensor tendons as in the forelimb.

Hind lower limb flexion

The muscles which flex the lower leg are not as obvious as in the forelimb because they lie under the muscles of the second thigh. They are the:

- Superficial digital flexor muscles
- Deep digital flexor muscles.

They are aided by the powerful gastrocnemius muscle that ends in the Achilles tendon running over the hock. The flexor muscles end in the flexor tendons which themselves attach to the pastern and pedal bones.

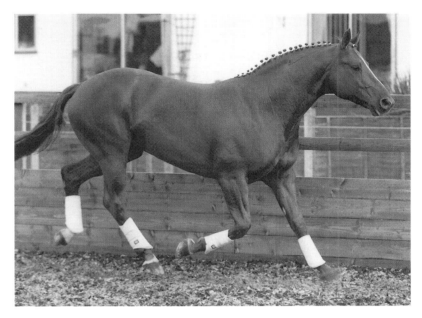

Fig. 9.20   Right hind and left fore impact

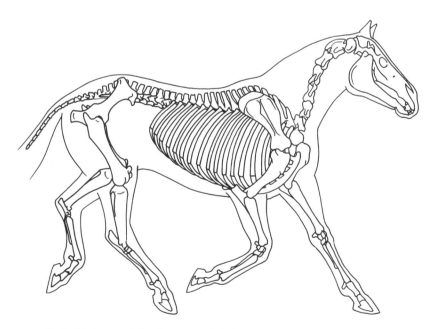

Fig. 9.21   Right hind and left fore impact – skeleton

The trot in dressage

The trot in dressage terms has four variations:

- Collected
- Working
- Medium
- Extended.

More advanced movements such as passage and piaffe are also variations of the trot. The regularity of the hoof beats of the diagonal legs, interrupted by the suspension phase, give rise to the rhythm of the trot. It is important that the rhythm stays the same in the variations of the trot. This is achieved by the top dressage horses by maintaining almost the same tempo in the transitions between collected, working, medium and extended trot. As the horse becomes more collected and the stride shortens, the legs will have to be lifted higher if the rhythm is to stay the same. These elevated steps give the trot *cadence*.

Collected trot

In the collected trot the hind feet usually step just short of the imprints left by the forefeet. The hindquarters are more engaged and the steps should be higher, rounder and more energetic. These elevated steps give the trot cadence. As the muscles that act as abdominal and hip flexors become stronger the hindquarters are drawn more underneath the horse and carry more weight. The horse's centre of gravity moves back, the forehand becomes lighter and the head and neck are carried higher, with the head close to the vertical.

Working trot

This is the horse's natural trot. With novice horses it is used to establish rhythm, balance, impulsion and strength. The hind feet step into or slightly beyond the hoof prints of the forefeet. The length of stride is 2.4–3 metres (8–9 feet).

Medium trot

In medium trot the stride is longer and more energetic than in working trot. The hind feet step beyond the hoof prints of the forefeet. The horse is allowed to lengthen the frame slightly and to carry the head and neck a little lower to allow greater freedom of the shoulders.

Extended trot

In extended trot the horse reaches maximum stride length with the hind feet stepping well in front of the hoof prints of the forefeet. There is greater power and engagement from the hindquarters to generate the necessary thrust.

The increased speed of the extended trot is a result of taking longer strides. Only a small part of the increase in stride length is due to a longer distance between the diagonal pair of limbs when they are on the ground. The majority of the increase in stride length is a result of more over tracking (the distance between the imprint of the front hoof and the subsequent imprint of the hind hoof on the same side), which is achieved as a result of a bigger suspension. The horse is propelled higher into the air, stays airborne longer, and covers a greater forward distance during the suspension period.

Freedom of the shoulder

For the horse to develop the medium and extended trot it must have free shoulder action. The biceps and the brachiocephalicus muscles contract to bring the horse's shoulder and forelimb forwards with simultaneous relaxation and stretching of the triceps muscle attached to the lower edge of the scapula. If the triceps muscle is unable to relax, the forward movement of the shoulder and hence the stride length will be inhibited. The horse's neck is lifted and hollowed by the contraction of the trapezius, serratus ventralis and rhomboideus muscles which attach to the top of the scapula: thus the contraction of these muscles holds the scapula and prevents the triceps from stretching, inhibits shoulder movement and prevents effective lengthening of the stride. When the horse's neck is flexed and stretched forwards, these muscles are relaxed and allow the triceps more freedom to stretch.

It should be remembered that:

- A horse that is tight and hollow in its neck will not be able to lengthen correctly.
- It is important to allow the horse to lengthen its frame slightly to attain a longer stride.
- Medium and extended trot demand power. Power is developed from collection. Medium trot should only be attempted when the horse has developed sufficient strength and collection.
- In practical terms, the development of collection and extension proceeds at the same time.

The ridden trot

Figures 9.22–9.24 show the ridden horse in right diagonal stance. This is equivalent to the moment in the stride shown in Fig. 9.2. The horse is showing a rounder outline and greater flexion of the knee and hock, indicating that the rider is helping to generate more impulsion. The rider is keeping an even and light contact on the rein, which allows the horse to carry his nose slightly in front of the vertical so the length of the stride has not been compromised or shortened. In rising trot on the right rein the rider sits on the right diagonal, when the left shoulder comes back and the inside hind leg is on the ground. This enables the rider to activate the inside hind leg and generate more energy and impulsion.

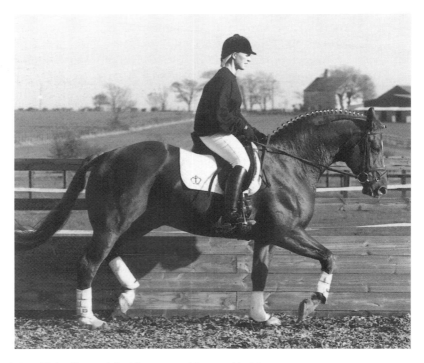

Fig. 9.22 Right diagonal double stance of horse with rider

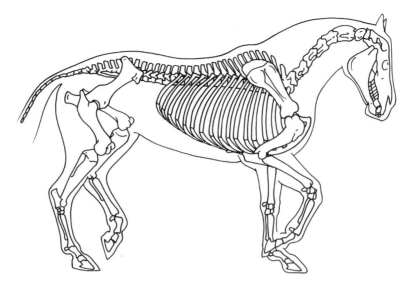

Fig. 9.23   Right diagonal double stance of ridden horse – skeleton

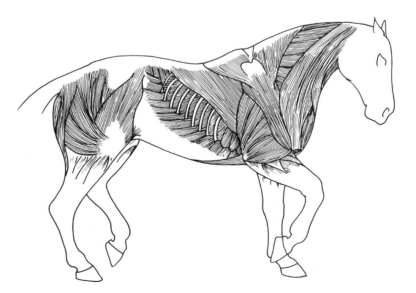

Fig. 9.24   Right diagonal double stance of ridden horse – musculature

The ridden trot – suspension

Figures 9.25–9.27 shows the suspension phase with rider, and is equivalent to the moment in the stride shown in Fig. 9.8. The young horse has responded to the demand of the rider by springing higher off the ground and taking a bigger step with the hind legs. Once the horse has been taught to take longer steps with the forelegs, it will be able to show impressive extensions. The horse needs to show a little more activity with the forelimbs as the front and hind feet are barely missing each other.

It is not easy for the rider to maintain the correct seat during the moment of suspension, so the trot places higher demands on the rider than the walk. Rising trot makes it easier for the rider to stay in balance with the horse during the suspension and relieves the horse's back of the rider's weight, giving the horse the freedom to move. It is generally easier for the horse to learn to lengthen the stride in trot if the rider is rising than if they are sitting.

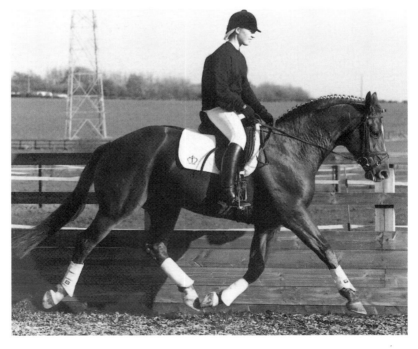

Fig. 9.25 First suspension phase of horse with rider

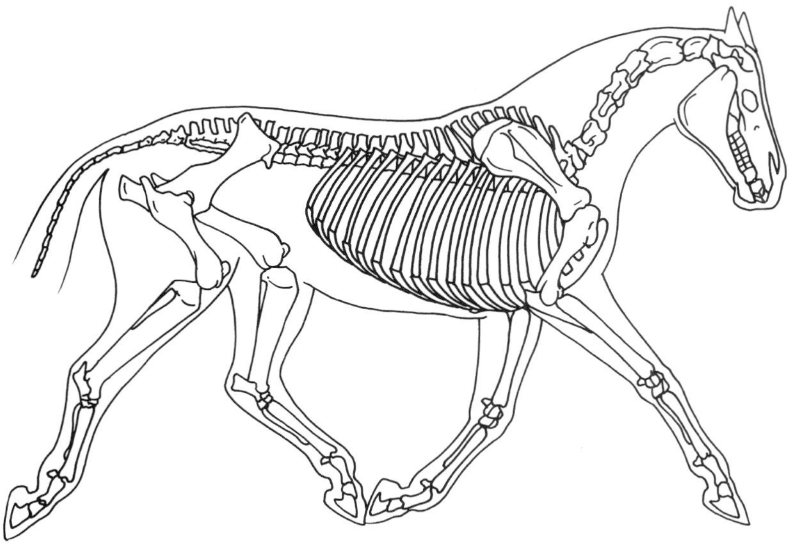

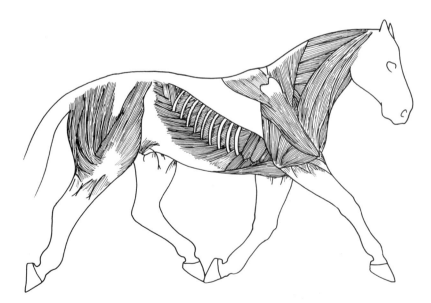

Fig. 9.26   First suspension phase of ridden horse – skeleton

Fig. 9.27   First suspension phase of ridden horse – musculature

Working trot

A forwards working trot like that shown in Fig. 9.25 covers about 220 metres per minute, and is the speed used in phases A and C (roads and tracks) of a three-day event. However, the speed of the trot can range between 160 and 280 metres per minute. The length of the stride in working trot is 2.4–3.0 metres (8–9 feet).

Lameness

Although the walk is useful for assessing a horse, it is the trot that is used to diagnose lameness. Indeed, much lameness is only visible in trot. During trot there should be four equal weight-bearing strides. If a horse is lame in front, it will nod its head as the sound leg hits the ground. This is because the horse is favouring the sound leg by placing more weight on it as it lands.

If hind limb lameness is suspected the horse should be observed for asymmetrical movement of the hindquarters, with the quarter of the lame leg appearing to rise and fall more than the other side.

Chapter 10

Cantering

Characteristics of the canter

Canter has the following characteristics:

- Medium speed gait
- The left and right sides move in different manners, with one side (left or right) trailing and one side leading, i.e. it is asymmetrical
- One diagonal limb pair moves more or less synchronously, with the trailing forelimb impacting before the leading hind limb
- Three-time beat
- There is a moment of suspension before the next stride.

Qualities of a good canter

A good canter should show the following characteristics:

- Light, with regular strides, good rhythm and balance.
- The hindquarters should be correctly engaged. This is shown by the horse carrying the hind limbs with adequate joint flexion and placing each hind foot on the ground firmly and with no hesitation.
- There should be a regular, three-time beat. The canter may become four-time when a horse is slowed down without sufficient impulsion but this is incorrect.
- The horse should be straight with the shoulders directly in front of the hindquarters.
- The head should move in co-ordination with the horizontal movement of the body.
- There should be a well-defined airborne phase when the horse is in gathered suspension, with all four feet off the ground.

Changing the lead

The canter is an asymmetrical gait; on the right rein the horse should canter on the right lead and on the left rein it should canter on the left lead.

When riding a young horse a change of canter lead can be made by bringing the horse back to trot, making a change of rein and re-establishing the new canter lead. As the horse becomes more educated, this change of lead can be made through walk. At higher levels of training horses are taught to make a flying change; the horse remains in canter and makes a change of lead during the suspension phase of the stride. Most horses, even when loose in the field, naturally canter on the correct lead for the direction in which they are travelling. Many horses also perform flying changes quite naturally as they change direction while cantering loose.

Footfall sequence of the canter

The footfall sequence for canter on a right lead is left hind, left (ipsilateral) fore and right (contralateral) hind together, right (ipsilateral) fore, followed by a suspension phase (Fig. 10.1).

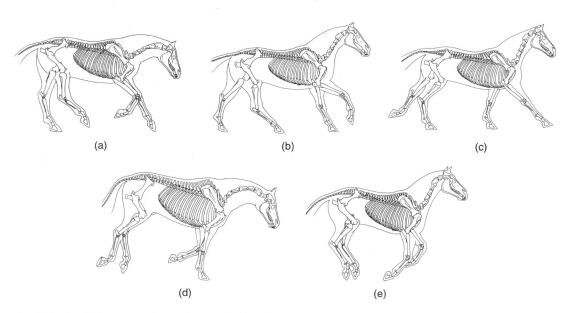

(a)   (b)   (c)

(d)   (e)

Fig. 10.1 Footfall sequence for canter on a right lead

Trailing hind single stance (Figs 10.2–10.4)

Fig. 10.2 shows the left hind in contact with the ground (because the horse is in right canter so the left hind is called the trailing limb). This part of the stride is known as the *trailing hind single stance* because the left hind is the only limb in contact with the ground. Note the position of the horse's head and neck as it rocks forwards in preparation for the left fore and right hind to hit the ground.

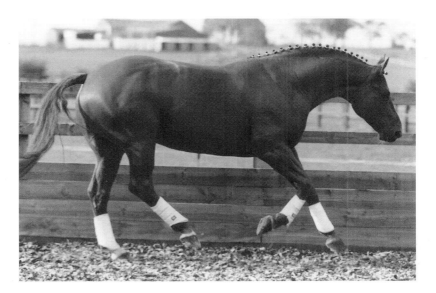

Fig. 10.2 Trailing (left) hind single stance

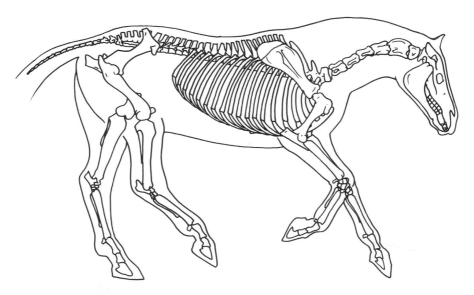

Fig. 10.3 Trailing (left) hind single stance – skeleton

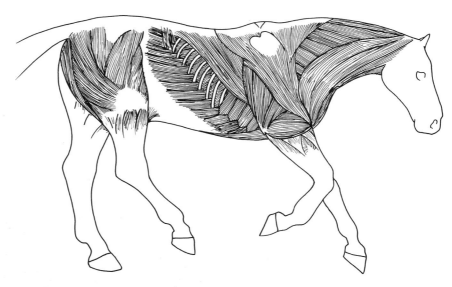

Fig. 10.4 Trailing (left) hind single stance – musculature

Hind tripedal stance (Figs 10.5–10.7)

In Fig. 10.5 the left fore and right hind have landed and the left hind has not yet been lifted, so the horse has three limbs in contact with the ground. This is known as the *hind tripedal stance*. As the horse is on the right lead, the right hind is called the *hind leading limb*. The neck and head are raised so that the centre of gravity has moved back and the horse carries more weight on the hind limbs (Fig. 10.2).

Balance and the centre of gravity

The horse is balanced when its weight is over its centre of gravity. Try balancing a ruler on the end of your finger. When you have manoeuvred the ruler so that it stays horizontal, you have found its centre of gravity. The centre of gravity in a standing horse is located around the 12th to 13th ribs, close to a line connecting the point of the shoulder with the point of buttock, more or less beneath the position of the rider's seat bones. When the horse is standing square its centre of gravity can be judged by drawing a chalk line from the point of the shoulder to the point of the buttocks, then counting forwards from the last (18th) rib. When you get to the space between the 12th and 13th ribs, follow the groove to the chalk line. The position of the centre of gravity varies with the individual horse and depends on its conformation and bodyweight. Because the centre of gravity lies nearer to the shoulder than to the hips the horse carries about two-thirds of its weight on its front legs. This is why many horses tend to fall onto their forehand.

As the position of the head and neck has a significant effect on the horse's balance and weight distribution the horse is able to alter the position of its centre of gravity by moving them. When the head and neck are lowered, more weight is carried on the front limbs and the horse's centre of gravity moves forward (Fig. 10.2). However, when the head and neck are raised, more weight is carried on the hind limbs and the centre of gravity moves back (Fig. 10.5).

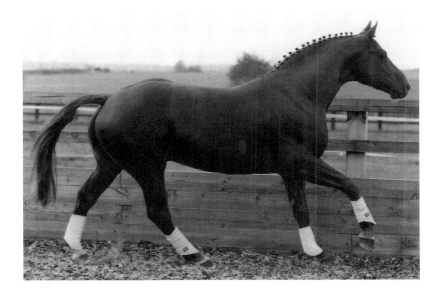

Fig. 10.5 Hind tripedal stance

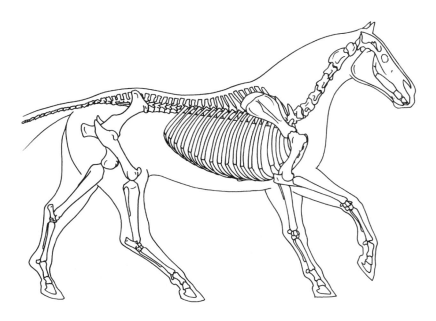

Fig. 10.6 Hind tripedal stance – skeleton

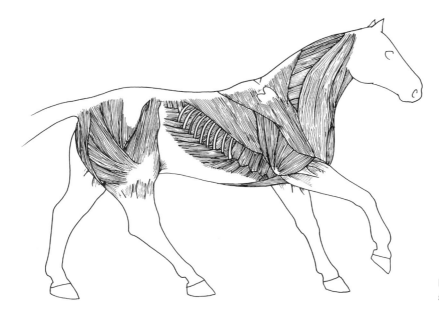

Fig. 10.7 Hind tripedal stance – musculature

Right diagonal double stance (Figs 10.8–10.10)

In Fig. 10.8 the left hind has left the ground but the right fore has not yet impacted. This leaves the horse with the right hind and left fore on the ground. This is known as the *right diagonal double stance*. The right (leading) fore then hits the ground so that the horse now has three legs on the ground: the right hind, left fore and right fore. This is known as the *fore tripedal stance*.

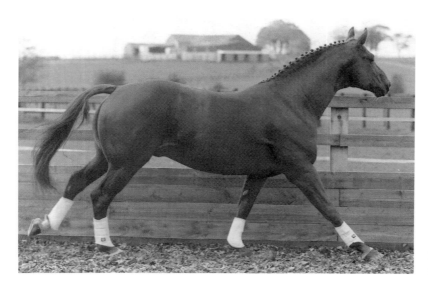

Fig. 10.8 Right diagonal double stance

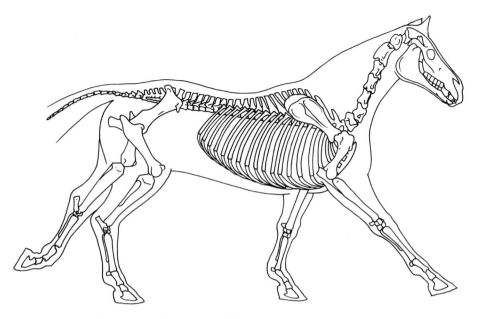

Fig. 10.9   Right diagonal double stance – skeleton

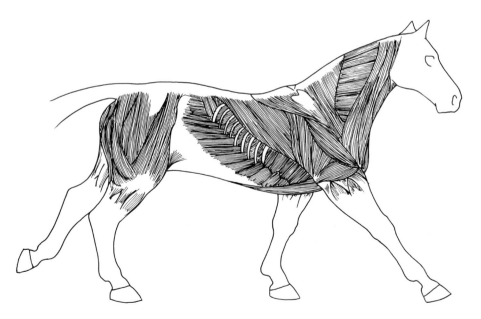

Fig. 10.10   Right diagonal double stance – musculature

Lead fore single stance (Figs 10.11–10.13)

The next limbs to leave the ground are the left fore and right hind, so that the horse has only the right fore on the ground. Note how the horse's head and neck have dropped as the hindquarters rise, propelling the horse forwards over the right fore which acts as a pivot.

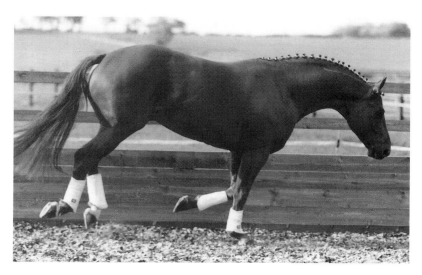

Fig. 10.11   Lead fore single stance

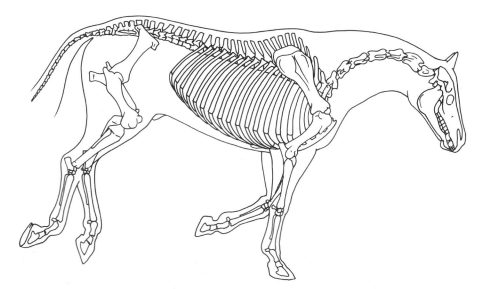

Fig. 10.12   Lead fore single stance – skeleton

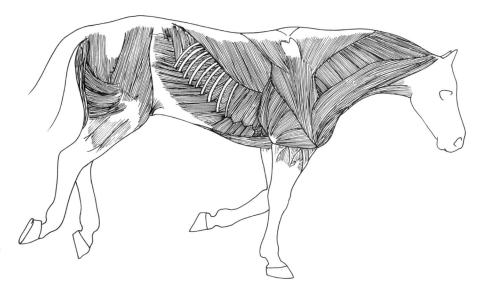

Fig. 10.13
Lead fore single
stance –
musculature

Gathered suspension phase (Figs 10.14–10.16)

The right fore pushes off the ground, bringing the forehand up, so that the horse moves into the *gathered suspension phase* (to differentiate it from the suspension phase seen in the trot). The hindquarters drop, the head rises and the left hind hits the ground to begin the next stride.

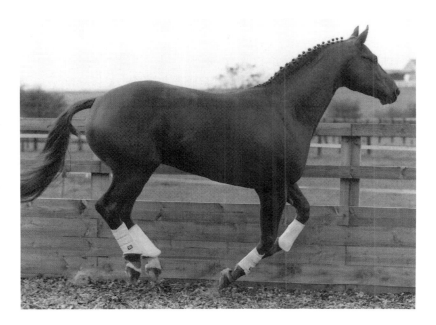

Fig. 10.14 Gathered
suspension phase

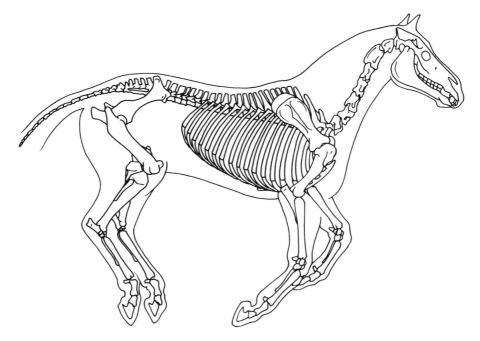

Fig. 10.15 Gathered suspension phase – skeleton

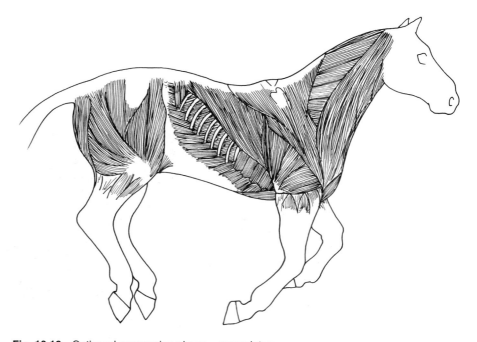

Fig. 10.16 Gathered suspension phase – musculature

The canter in dressage

The following canters are recognised in dressage terms:

- Collected
- Working
- Medium.

One of the aims of dressage training is to change the horse's balance by shifting more weight onto the hindquarters, allowing the forehand to become lighter and more mobile. When the trained horse carries itself in a collected outline, the hindquarters are lowered and the neck is raised.

Counter canter

Counter canter is used as an exercise to improve suppleness in the shoulders and back. The rider asks the horse to lead with the outside forelimb instead of the inside; on a circle to the left the horse canters with the right lead, with the bend over the leading leg. A disunited canter is incorrect and occurs when the forehand is on one lead and the hindquarters on another.

Cantering with rider

Left hind single stance (Figs 10.17–10.19)

Figure 10.17 shows canter on a right lead with a rider. This is equivalent to the part of the stride shown in Fig. 10.2. The left hind is the only limb

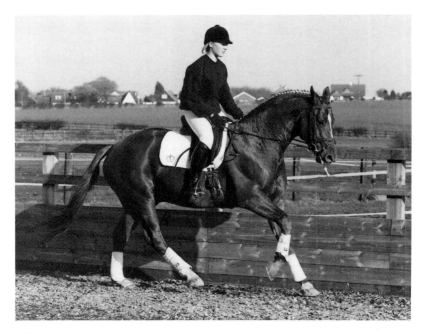

Fig. 10.17 Left hind single stance of horse with rider

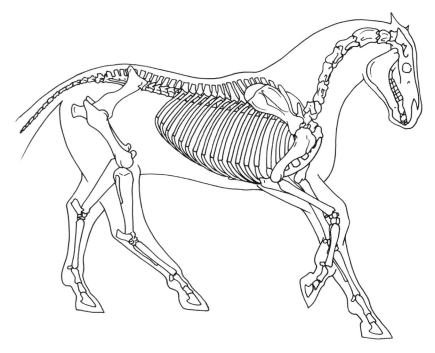

Fig. 10.18   Left hind single stance of ridden horse – skeleton

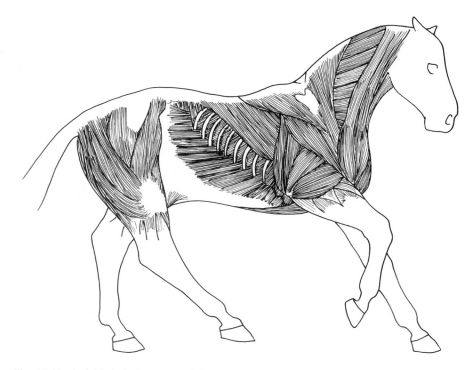

Fig. 10.19   Left hind single stance of ridden horse – musculature

in contact with the ground. The horse has responded to the rider by bringing its nose back to the vertical and shortening its neck slightly, so moving its centre of gravity back. To remain balanced the horse must engage its hindquarters and bring its right hind further under its body than seen in Fig. 10.2.

Hind tripedal stance (Figs 10.20, 10.21)

Figure 10.20 shows the equivalent stage of the stride to Fig. 10.5. The left fore and right hind have landed together, and the left hind has not yet been lifted. The right hind is further under the horse's body than in Fig. 10.5, giving it greater impulsion. The horse has not achieved the same degree of elevation of the right forelimb, suggesting that its forehand is not as fully developed as its hindquarters.

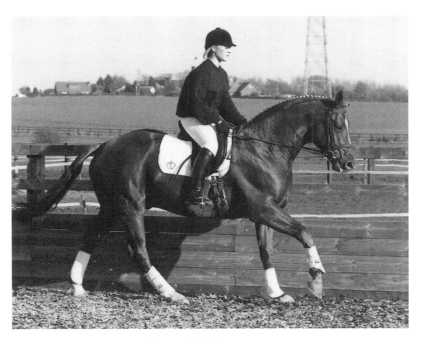

Fig. 10.20   Hind tripedal stance of horse with rider

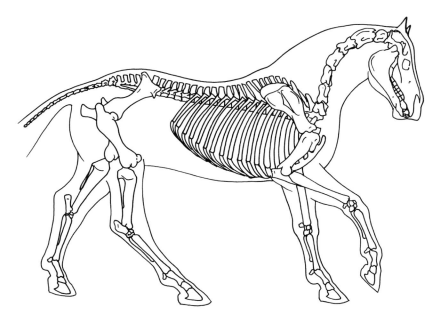

Fig. 10.21 Hind tripedal stance of ridden horse – skeleton

The next stance is the right diagonal double stance, and this is discussed on page 135.

Right diagonal double stance (Figs 10.22–10.24)

Figure 10.22 shows the equivalent part of the stride to Fig. 10.8. The left hind has left the ground but the right fore has not yet impacted. The right (leading) fore is fully extended before hitting the ground and initial contact will be slightly 'heel first'. The greater engagement of the hindquarters is demonstrated by the positioning of the right hind in advance of a line dropped from the stifle. The degree of stress placed on the pastern and fetlock, even at this relatively slow speed is also apparent. The importance of adequate slope to the shoulder is emphasised by its limiting effect on the amount of reach that the right fore can achieve. A rider who inhibits the horse's ability to lengthen the neck will also limit the length of stride of the forelimb.

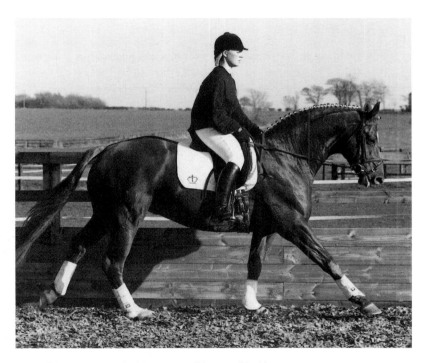

Fig. 10.22   Right diagonal double stance of horse with rider

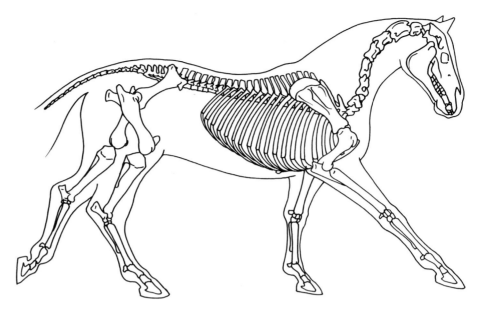

Fig. 10.23   Right diagonal double stance of ridden horse – skeleton

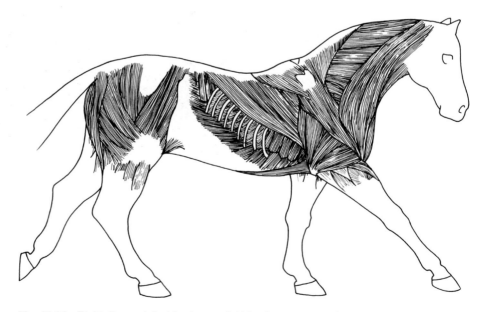

Fig. 10.24   Right diagonal double stance of ridden horse – musculature

Lead fore single stance (Figs 10.25–10.27)

Figure 10.25 shows an equivalent stage in the horse's stride to that shown in Fig. 10.11. The left fore and the right hind have left the ground leaving the horse with only the right forelimb on the ground. The greater engagement of the hindquarters and the fact that the centre of gravity is further back, mean that the horse does not have to use its head and neck to balance itself to the same extent. The position of the rider is also keeping the weight off the horse's forehand and allowing it to balance effectively.

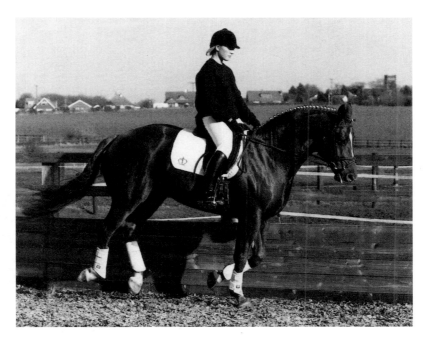

Fig. 10.25 Lead fore single stance of horse with rider

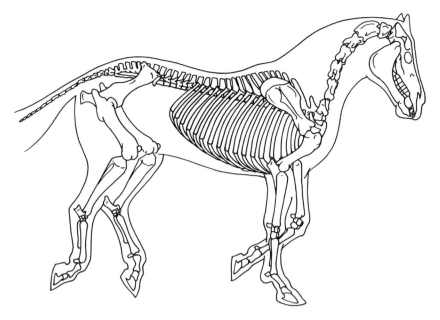

Fig. 10.26   Lead fore single stance of ridden horse – skeleton

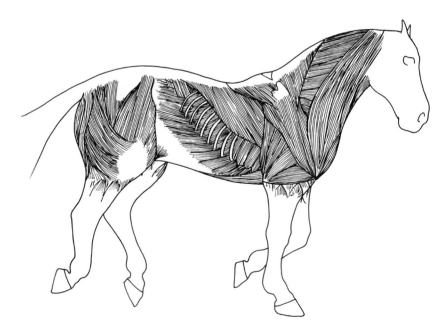

Fig. 10.27   Lead fore single stance of ridden horse – musculature

Gathered suspension phase (Figs 10.28, 10.29)

Figure 10.28 shows the equivalent stage in the stride to Fig. 10.14, with the horse in gathered suspension. While the hindquarters are more engaged, there appears to be less lift in the horse's forelimbs.

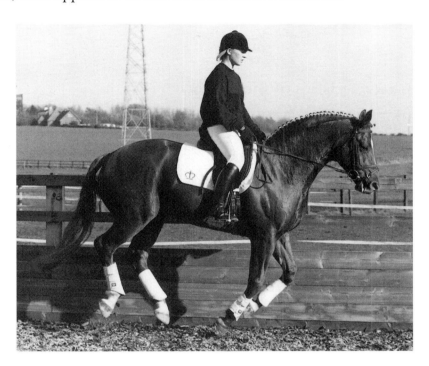

Fig. 10.28 Gathered suspension phase of horse with rider

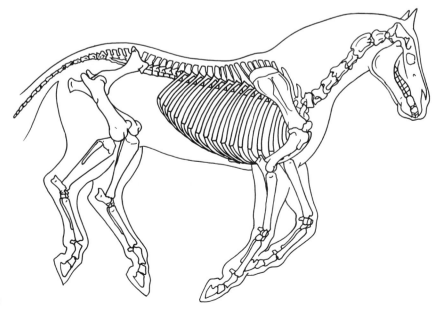

Fig. 10.29 Gathered suspension phase of ridden horse – skeleton

Chapter 11

Galloping

Characteristics of the gallop

The gallop has the following features:

- High speed
- Asymmetrical
- Four-time beat
- Non-lead hind, lead hind, non-lead fore, lead fore
- One airborne phase per stride.

The gallop consists of a series of springs through the air during which the horse never has more than two feet on the ground at once and usually only one.

Coupling of respiration and stride rates

The respiratory rate is linked to the horse's gait, and at gallop the stride rate equals the respiration rate. This known as locomotory–respiratory coupling and its purpose is to ensure that the muscles of breathing and movement do not work against each other. As the galloping horse lifts its forelimbs, the head is raised, the gut moves back and the horse breathes in. As the forelimbs hit the ground, the head drops, the gut moves forwards, helping the horse to breathe out.

Dynamic equilibrium

When a horse is moving it is said to be in *dynamic equilibrium*. This means that the horse keeps its balance because as its body falls towards the centre of gravity another limb is placed on the ground which 'catches' the horse's weight, supports the body and projects it forwards.

The faster the horse is moving, the more it will rely on dynamic equilibrium to stay upright. The slower the gait the greater the need for more support. This is achieved by having more feet in contact with the ground. A good way to understand balance is to think about riding a bicycle: as you cycle along at a reasonable speed it is easy to keep your balance but the slower you go the harder this becomes. Eventually, when the bicycle comes to a stop, it will topple to one side unless you put a foot on the ground to increase the area of support. Similarly, horses do very well with only one or two feet on the ground during the gallop, but an increase in the number of supporting feet is needed in the slower gaits.

Changing the lead

Like the canter, the gallop is an asymmetrical gait and the horse gallops on either the left or right lead. In most competitions where the horse is galloping there is no requirement to change lead; races are run in straight lines or on circular tracks. In long distance races horses will perform a flying change of lead. A tired horse will change lead more frequently than one that is less fatigued.

Footfall sequence of the gallop

The gallop is the fastest quadrupedal gait. The left and right sides move in different manners, with one side (left or right) trailing and one side leading. The four limbs move individually and the sequence of footfalls is: non-lead hind, lead hind, non-lead fore, lead fore (Fig. 11.1). So for a right lead gallop the sequence would be left hind, right hind, left fore, right fore.

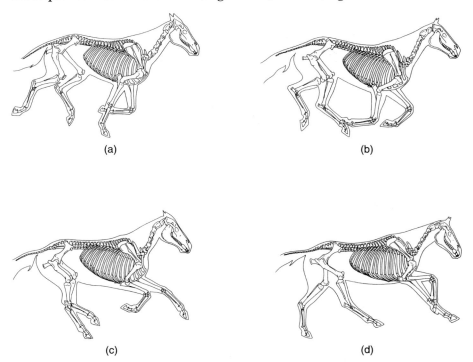

(a)   (b)

(c)   (d)

Fig. 11.1 Footfall sequence of the gallop

Non-lead (left) fore lift-off (Figs 11.2–11.4)

Figure 11.2 shows the left fore lift-off from the ground. As the horse is on the right lead this is called the non-lead fore lift-off. The horse has only the right fore on the ground and is said to be in *lead fore single stance*. The horse's body is launched off the ground by a powerful thrust of the leading forelimb, marking the end of fore lead single stance and the start of the airborne phase in gathered suspension.

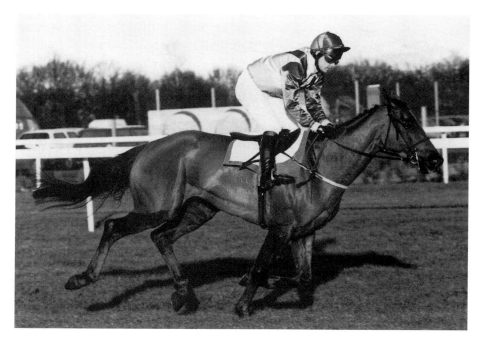

Fig. 11.2   Left fore lift-off

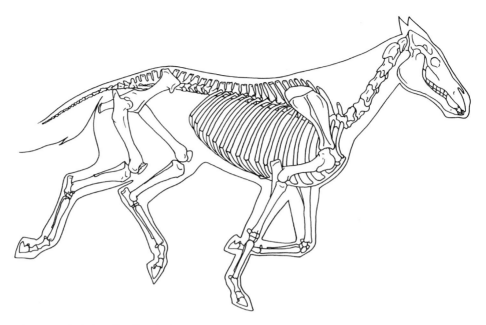

Fig. 11.3   Left fore lift-off – skeleton

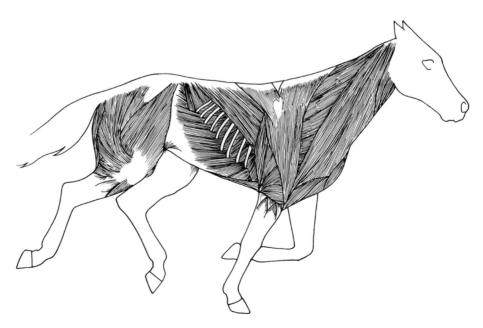

Fig. 11.4   Left fore lift-off – musculature

Suspension phase (Figs 11.5–11.7)

Figure 11.5 shows the airborne phase of the stride with the horse in gathered suspension. In a galloping horse the forelimbs are just as responsible for propulsion as the hindquarters. The suspension phase allows the horse to:

- Recover its equilibrium – in lead fore single stance (Fig. 11.2) the horse's centre of gravity has shifted forwards and the viscera have pressed against the lungs, forcing the horse to breathe out. The horse needs to move the centre of gravity back again to be able to inhale. Respiration rates can reach 180 breaths per minute.
- Get its hind feet underneath the body – the combination of body weight and a rigid spine mean that if a foreleg was on the ground the horse would not be able to bring the hind limbs sufficiently underneath the body. This contrasts with the greyhound, which has a flexible spine, which enables it to get its hind limbs right under its body.

In the gallop the spine can be flexed slightly to bring the hind limbs forward at the beginning of the stride. The croup is flexed (Fig. 11.6) around the lumbosacral joint by contraction of the hip flexors (psoas major and iliacus) and relaxation of the longissimus dorsi and middle gluteal muscles. Sideways movement of the spine is minimised by the iliocostalis, longissimus, spinalis and multifidus muscles.

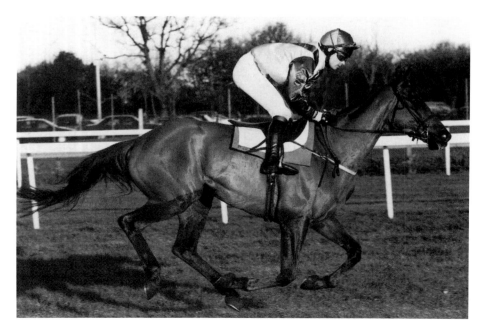

Fig. 11.5
Suspension phase

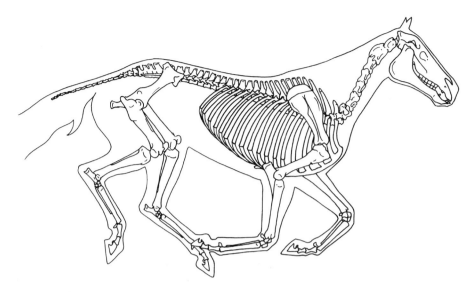

Fig. 11.6   Suspension phase – skeleton

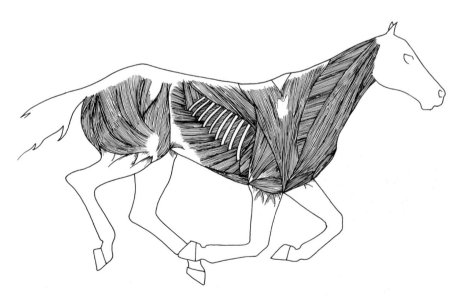

Fig. 11.7   Suspension phase – musculature

Non-lead (left) hind impact (Figs 11.8–11.10)

In Fig. 11.8 the non-lead (left) hind is about to hit the ground. During this phase it is the only foot on the ground so this is known as the *non-lead hind single stance*.

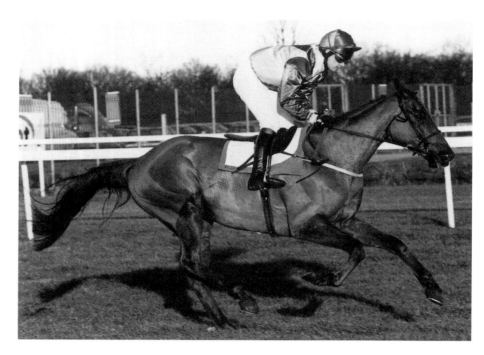

Fig. 11.8 Non-lead (left) hind impact

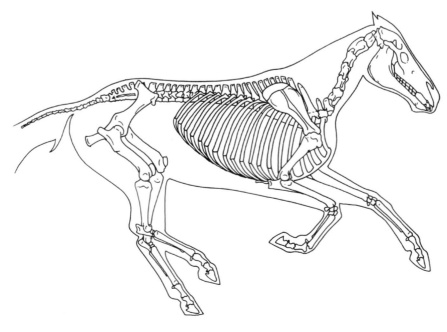

Fig. 11.9 Non-lead (left) hind impact – skeleton

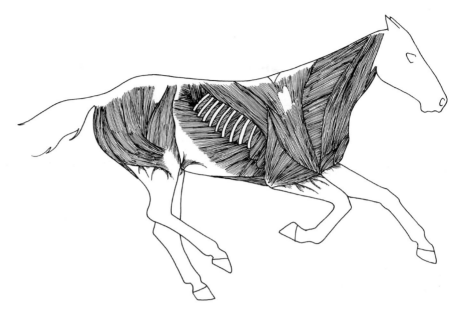

Fig. 11.10 Non-lead (left) hind impact – musculature

Lead (right) hind impact (Figs 11.11–11.13)

Figure 11.11 shows the moment before lead (right) hind limb impact. This will mark the end of the non-lead single stance and the start of the hind double stance, in which both hind feet are in contact with the ground.

When the foot contacts the ground the lumbosacral curve flattens (Fig. 11.12) through the action of the horse's body weight and contraction of the longissimus dorsi and middle gluteal muscles (Fig. 11.13). This flexion is limited and the muscles work together to keep the spine as rigid as possible.

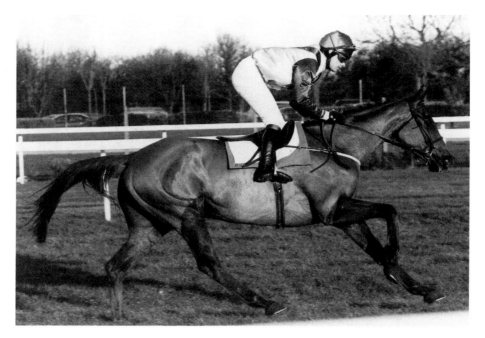

Fig. 11.11   Lead (right) hind impact

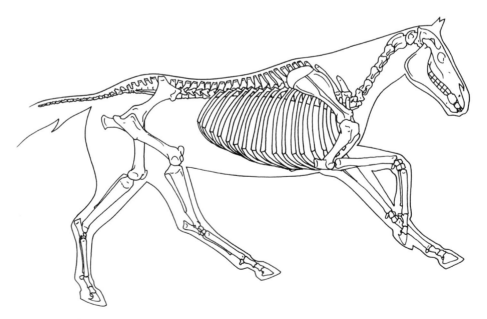

Fig. 11.12   Lead (right) hind impact – skeleton

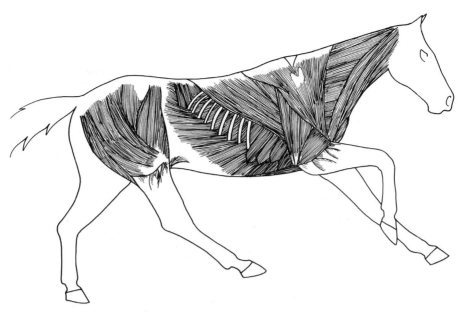

Fig. 11.13   Lead (right) hind impact – musculature

Subsequent footfall sequence

The lead (right) hind impact is followed by:

- Non-lead (left) hind lift-off. This leavies the horse with only the right hind on the ground (*lead hind single stance*).
- Non-lead (left) fore impact. This marks the end of lead hind single stance and the start of *right diagonal double stance*. The horse has the right hind and left fore on the ground.
- Lead (right) hind lift-off. This ends the right diagonal double stance and marks the start of *non-lead fore single stance*.
- Lead (right) fore impact. This ends the non-lead fore single stance and marks the start of *fore double stance*, during which the horse is supported only by both front limbs.
- The non-lead (left) hind will then hit the ground, marking the start of the subsequent stride.

Role of the hind limbs

During the gallop the hind feet are driven powerfully against the ground. The shorter the period between the hind feet contacting the ground, the more effectively they propel the horse. However, this also limits the time that one or both hind limbs can support the body. To counter this, the time between the two forelimbs making contact with the ground is maximised to support the horse's body as long as possible and over a greater distance as possible.

Stride length

The galloping horse may be able to extend a hind foot as far forwards as the umbilicus (mid-belly). The forefoot is unlikely to extend further forwards than the nose. However, Fig. 11.12 shows that the foot does not contact the ground until retraction (the limb moving back) is well underway. Propulsion does not occur until the body has passed over the vertical and the toe drives against the ground. The forefoot usually lands on the heel, while in a fast gallop little more than the toe of the hind foot makes ground contact.

Angulation of the hock

To produce maximum drive the toe of the hind foot should rotate through an arc as it leaves the ground. The power is then transferred directly to the hindquarters, to the pelvis, through the spine and thus to the forehand. A sickle hock with too much angulation will result in a longer stride. A horse that is straighter through the hock has a limb that swings more naturally from the hip, like a pendulum, and allows more frequent strides. Thoroughbreds that are bred to sprint are frequently straight limbed and can outrun a 'stayer' with a more angulated hock. However, the 'stayer' tends to perform better over a distance where a longer stride is more important than speed.

The dressage horse, with a strong, well angulated hock, will be able to flex the hock more easily and achieve more collection.

Warming the horse up and down

The horse must be thoroughly warmed up before being galloped; ideally, this should consist of 20–30 minutes walk, trot and canter. Race horses walk around the paddock, canter down to the start and then walk before the start of the race, ensuring that they are well prepared. The purpose of warming a horse up is to ensure that the blood carries nutrients deep into the muscles and that the nervous, hormonal, respiratory and muscular systems involved with exertion are primed. Horses that have been insufficiently warmed up are more susceptible to tendon, ligament and muscle injury, and will fatigue more rapidly.

Warming (or cooling) down is equally important to the horse's health and fitness. After exertion the horse should be kept moving (walk and gentle jog) until its respiration and heart rate have returned to normal. This may take up to 20 minutes after a race or cross country event. The galloping horse generates potential toxins as the result of anaerobic energy production, so warming down by keeping the horse moving ensures that the heart still pumps blood to the muscles at a relatively high rate. This gives the horse's body time to remove these substances from the muscles. If horses are cooled down too quickly these toxins may be left in the muscles, leading to stiffness and poor recovery from exertion.

Tips for the rider about safe galloping surfaces

Galloping on poor ground is a contributory factor to horses sustaining tendon and ligament injuries. Deep, hard, uneven, inconsistent and slippery ground is not suitable for galloping. If a horse's foot hits a soft patch or a rut or the foot slides unexpectedly, the muscles are unable to protect the tendons, a tendon may be overloaded and fibres within it may rupture and tear. The situation will be exacerbated if the horse is fatigued or if it has not been warmed up sufficiently.

Chapter 12

Jumping

The horse is not a natural jumper because of the relative rigidity of the spine, the heavy gut and large head.

Sequence of the jump

The sequence of the jump shown in Fig. 12.1 can be divided into five phases:

- Approach
- Take-off
- Airborne
- Landing
- Getaway.

Approach phase (Figs 12.2–12.8)

During the approach at the canter (Figs 12.2 and 12.5) the horse sees, appraises and accepts the fence. During the last three strides the horse lowers and stretches out its head and neck, enabling it to use its forehand to lift and round the back and also to bring the hind legs well under the body to aid propulsion over the fence. The last canter stride before the fence is different from the previous strides, as the horse prepares to take off, its head, neck and shoulders are lowered to allow the forelimbs to stretch out further. The higher the jump, the more the forelimbs must reach forward and the more the body is lowered to allow the hind limbs to come under the body and propel the horse upwards and over the jump (Fig. 12.6).

In Fig. 12.6 the rider has allowed the horse to take her hand and arm forwards and has kept her upper body fairly upright as the horse prepares to take off. This allows the horse to keep the head and neck in the natural position shown by the loose jumping horse (Fig. 12.5).

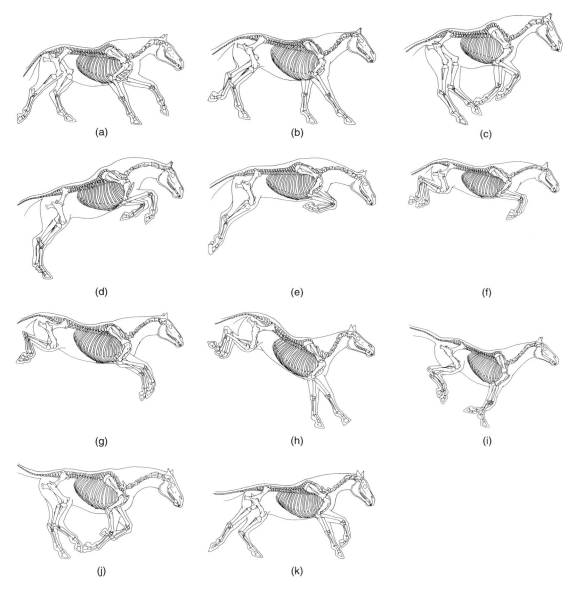

(a)

(b)

(c)

(d)

(e)

(f)

(g)

(h)

(i)

(j)

(k)

Fig. 12.1 Sequence of the jump

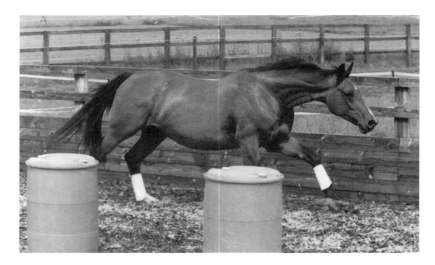

Fig. 12.2   Penultimate stride before take-off

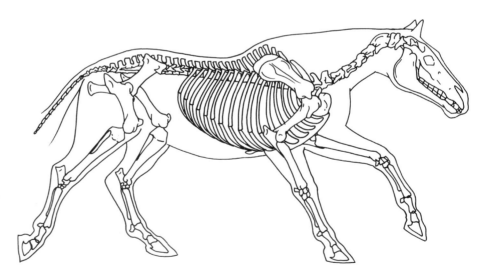

Fig. 12.3   Penultimate stride before take-off – skeleton

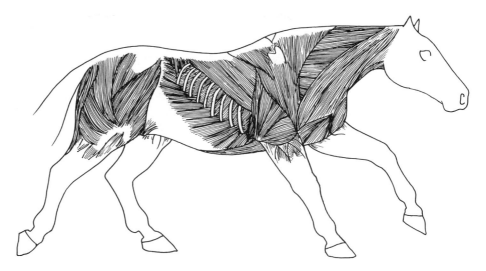

Fig. 12.4   Penultimate stride before take-off – musculature

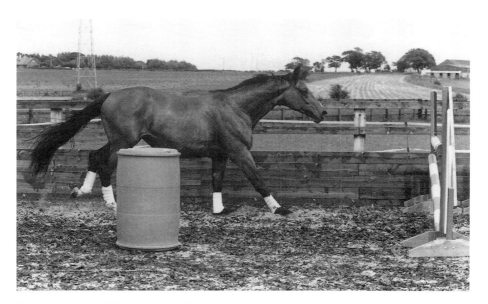

Fig. 12.5   Last stride before take-off

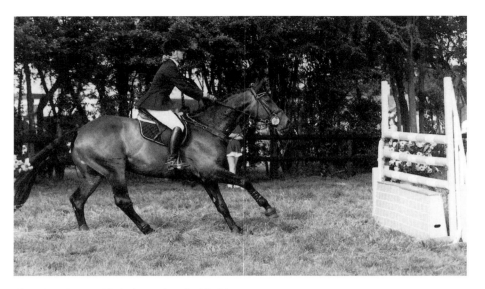

Fig. 12.6   Last stride before take-off with rider

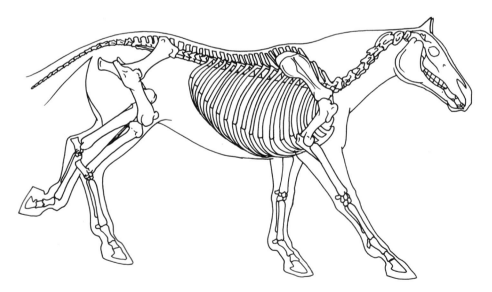

Fig. 12.7   Last stride before take-off – skeleton

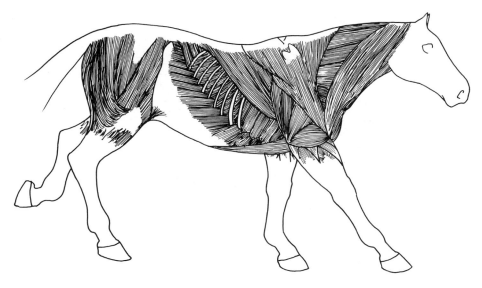

Fig. 12.8   Last stride before take-off – musculature

Take-off (Figs 12.9–12.16)

The lead (right) forelimb is the first to take off. The horse is then supported by the leading forelimb which straightens to push the front end into the air (Figs 12.9 and 12.10). Take-off ends at the lift-off of the lead hind limb. To lift the forehand off the ground, the horse has to move the centre of gravity backwards (the experienced jumper does this by raising his head and neck) as well as flexing the hocks.

In Fig. 12.10 the horse raises its head to enable the forelimbs to leave the ground. The rider has brought her hands back and inclined her upper body forwards, closing the angle of the elbow and maintaining a contact on the horse's mouth. Compared with the loose jumping horse (Fig. 12.9) this appears to have constrained the position of the horse's head and neck.

Role of the forelimbs in the take-off
The forelimbs play a very important role in the take-off, acting as struts that change forward momentum into the upward thrust of the forehand. This is clearly shown in Figs 12.9 and 12.10. The shoulder and the elbow are extended by the action of the triceps on the elbow joint, and by the biceps brachii and the supraspinatus on the shoulder joint. A large part of the impetus that pushes the horse upwards comes from the extension of the fetlock joint, brought about by the superficial and deep digital flexors. The muscles along the topline of the back, from the neck to the croup also contract, arching the back as much as possible and helping to lift the forehand (Fig. 12.12).

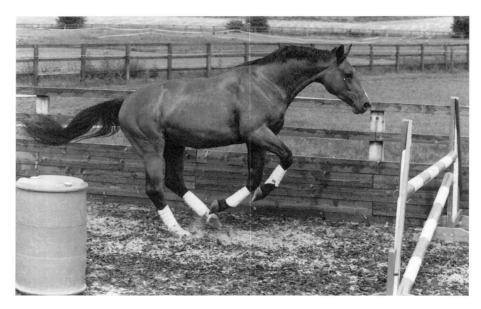

Fig. 12.9 Beginning take-off

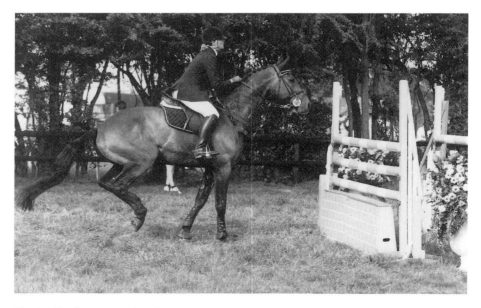

Fig. 12.10 Beginning take-off with rider

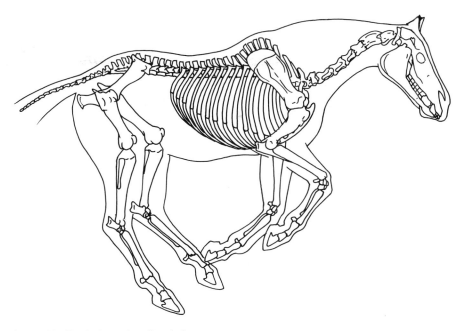

Fig. 12.11   Beginning take-off – skeleton

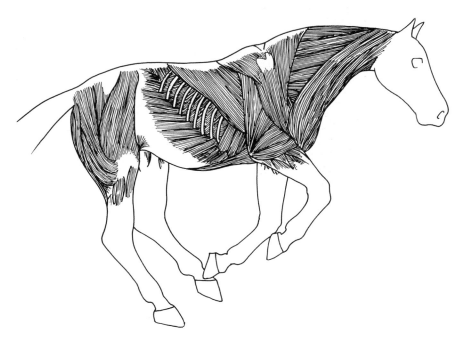

Fig. 12.12   Beginning take-off – musculature

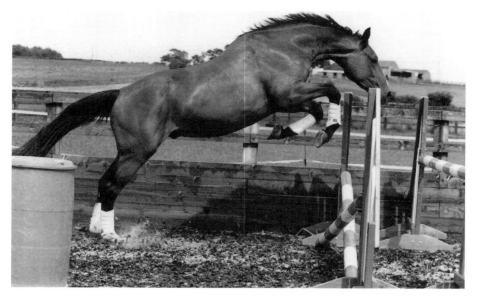

Fig. 12.13 Ending take-off

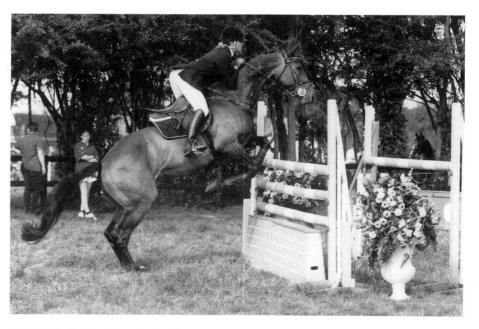

Fig. 12.14 Ending take-off with rider

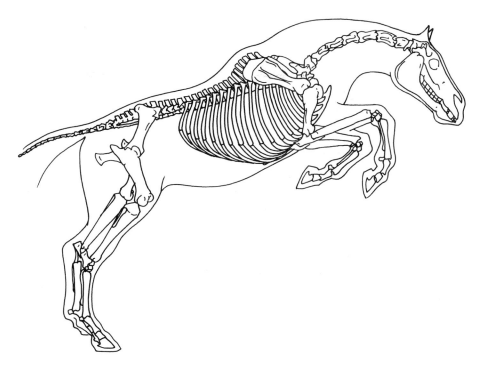

Fig. 12.15   Ending take-off – skeleton

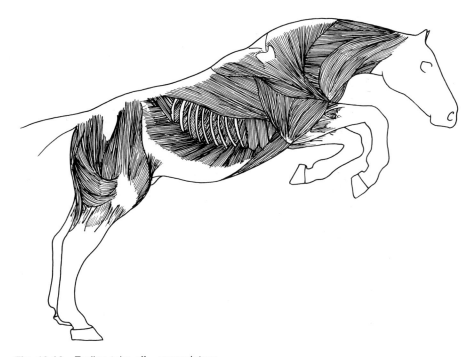

Fig. 12.16   Ending take-off – musculature

Role of the hindquarters in the take-off
As the horse's front end rises from the ground, the hindquarters rotate under the body to support its body weight (Fig. 12.14). The hind limbs push off close to the hoof print left by the leading forelimb. The hind limbs are not placed down exactly together (Fig. 12.9) and they do not leave the ground quite together. However, they do appear to be used more in unison in show jumping than when the horse is jumping at speed. The amount the forehand is elevated before take-off influences the trajectory through the air, while increased flexion of the hind limbs increases upwards impulsion.

Straightening the hind limbs
The horse drives its hind feet against the ground, straightening the hips, stifle, hocks and fetlocks (Figs 12.13 and 12.14). This results in the hindquarters and thighs travelling much faster than the lower limbs because the feet remain firmly on the ground until they are lifted by the movement of the body. The hip is extended by the hamstring group of muscles (biceps femoris, semitendinosus and semimembranosus muscles), aided by muscles attaching to the point of hip and the femur. The muscles of the quarters also extend the stifle and hock joints – stifle extension is aided by the quadriceps femoris, and hock extension is backed up by the gastrocnemius muscle (Fig. 12.16). The fetlock joint is straightened by the action of the deep digital flexor muscle.

Folding of the fore limbs
As soon as the front feet leave the ground, the forelimbs begin to flex, especially at the elbow and knee (Figs 12.9, 12.13, 12.14). This folding is helped by contraction of the brachiocephalicus muscle which brings the forelimbs upwards and forwards.

Airborne phase (Figs 12.17–12.28)

The trajectory, impulsion and speed determine the flight over the jump. Most of the joints in the horse's fore and hind limbs are flexed as the horse is propelled over the fence (Figs 12.21 and 12.22). The hind limbs can be flexed to bring the limbs underneath the body or extended behind the horse (Figs 12.25 and 12.26) in preparation for landing.

The classic parabola over a fence occurs when the horse slightly rounds its back and reaches to get over the fence. The more the horse can use its back, shoulders and hips the better. The less the limbs are flexed, the higher the horse must lift its body to clear the fence; a good showjumper uses limb flexion to full advantage. Some horses kick out behind the body to clear the fence, mainly through the action of the gastrocnemius muscle.

As the horse leaves the ground the rider should give it enough rein to allow the horse to lower its head and bring its withers up. The loose jumping horse in Fig. 12.17 shows the extent to which this may occur, while the ridden horse in Fig. 12.18 is not using its neck and shoulders with nearly as much freedom. The rider maintaining too short a rein while jumping is a common cause of a horse hitting a fence.

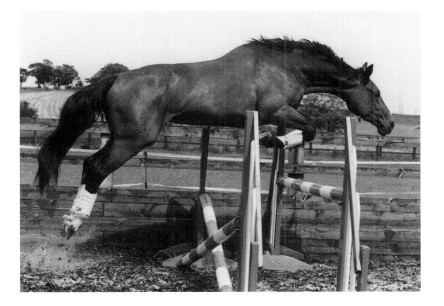

Fig. 12.17 First part of airborne phase

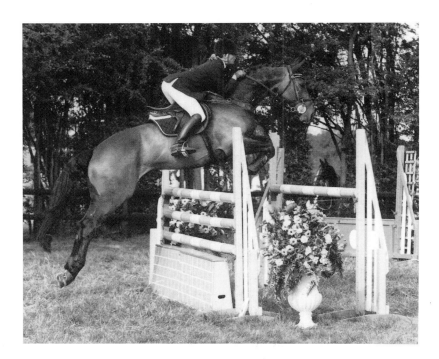

Fig. 12.18 First part of airborne phase with rider

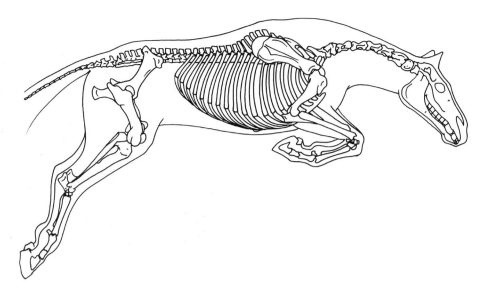

Fig. 12.19   First part of airborne phase – skeleton

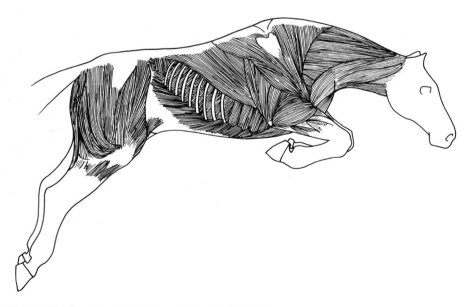

Fig. 12.20   First part of airborne phase – musculature

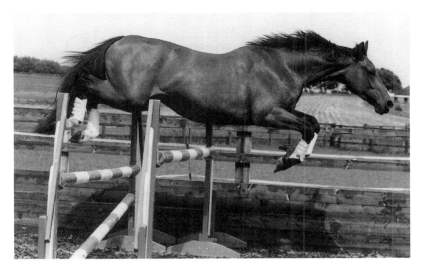

Fig. 12.21 Middle part of airborne phase

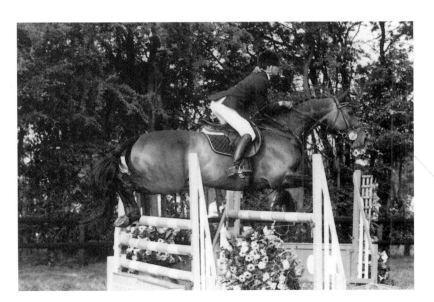

Fig. 12.22 Middle part of airborne phase with rider

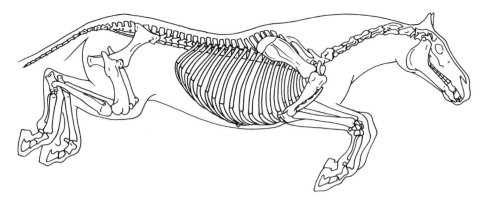

Fig. 12.23 Middle part of airborne phase – skeleton

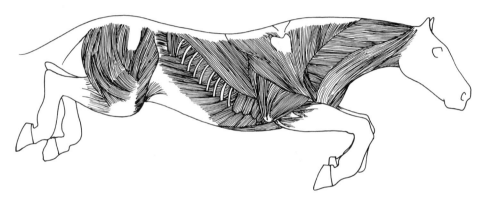

Fig. 12.24 Middle part of airborne phase – musuculature

Preparation for landing

Horse: at the same time that the hocks are flexing, the forelimbs extend in preparation for landing (Figs 12.25 and 12.26). The horse begins to raise the head and neck, shifting the centre of gravity back.

Rider: the rider has begun to bring her upper body back (Fig. 12.26) because moving her centre of gravity back will help her balance when the horse decelerates as it hits the ground. She has also begun to open the angle of the elbow, allowing the horse a little more freedom of the head and neck.

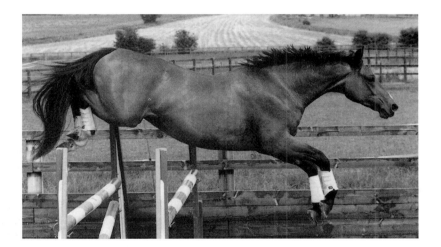

Fig. 12.25 Last part of airborne phase: descent

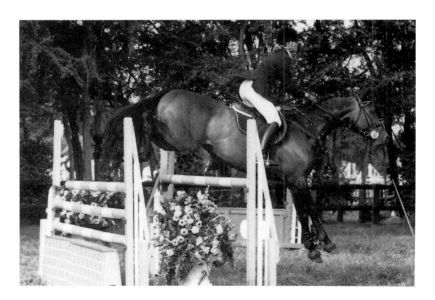

Fig. 12.26 Last part of airborne phase with rider: descent

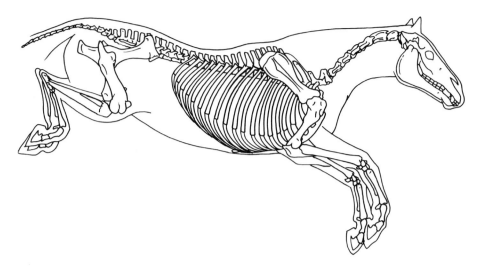

Fig. 12.27 Last part of airborne phase: descent – skeleton

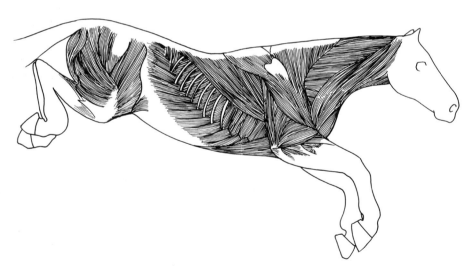

Fig. 12.28 Last part of airborne phase: descent – musculature

Landing (Figs 12.29–12.40)

One extended forelimb lands first, closely followed by the other, which is placed in front of the first to give a good base of support. Both the horses in Figs 12.29 and 12.30 demonstrate good use of the back and hips, ensuring that the hind feet clear the jump. The ridden horse (Fig. 12.30) has tilted the hindquarters to the left in its effort to clear the fence. The rider has opened his fingers on the rein, maintaining contact but allowing plenty of freedom while staying in balance with the horse.

On landing the forelimbs act as struts and the hind limbs are brought down under the body independently, not as a pair (Figs 12.29, 12.30, 12.33 and 12.34).

The loose jumping horse in Fig. 12.29 demonstrates how the non-lead (left) forelimb is used on landing as a strut for the forehand to pass over, before the lead (right) forelimb lands. The ridden horse in Fig. 12.30 shows the stress placed on the landing leg with over-extension of the fetlock joint and pressure on the front of the knee joint. The small bones of the knee are susceptible to chip fractures when placed under this type of extreme pressure.

The first limb to land is moved quickly out of the way to allow the hind limbs to land. In Fig. 12.33 the horse has already lifted the left fore. The hind limbs come down one after the other, but before the second has touched down, the forelimb has already pushed off. In Fig. 12.37 the left hind touches down first and the right fore is lifted, leaving the horse with all the weight on the left hind. The toe of the right hind coming down narrowly misses the toe of the right fore as it is being lifted. It is easy to understand why horses over reach in heavy going that delays the lift-off the forelimb.

Fig. 12.38 shows the period when the right hind has landed but the left fore has not yet left the ground. The position of the left hind demonstrates clearly why this horse has to wear over-reach boots.

If the forelimb is too far ahead on landing, the heel will contact the ground first, with the toe turning upwards, putting strain on the flexor tendons. With the limb too far ahead, it cannot be used as a pivot for the body to pass over it. To save itself from falling, the horse must bring its other forefoot forwards rapidly. Often the body sinks in front so that the other forelimb is unable to straighten in time, and the horse falls.

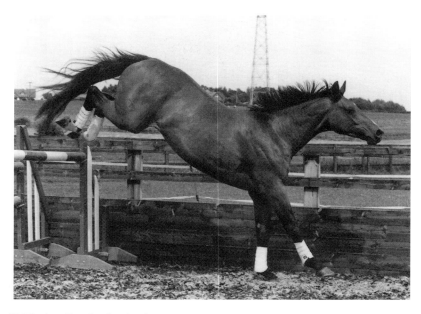

Fig. 12.29 Landing: leading leg impact

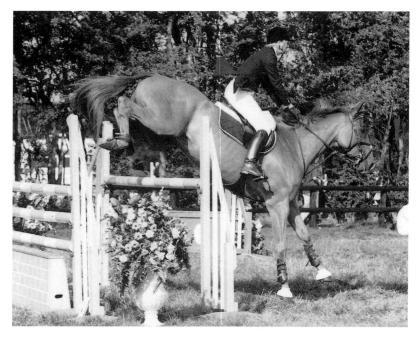

Fig. 12.30 Landing with rider: leading leg impact

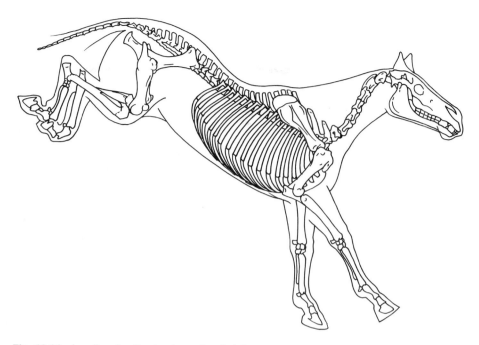

Fig. 12.31   Landing: leading leg impact – skeleton

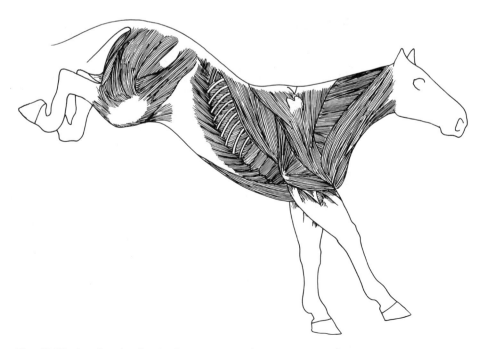

Fig. 12.32   Landing: leading leg impact – musculature

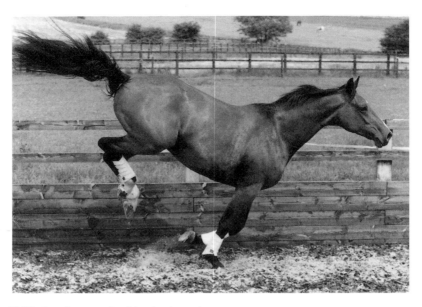

Fig. 12.33 Landing: non-lead foreleg impact

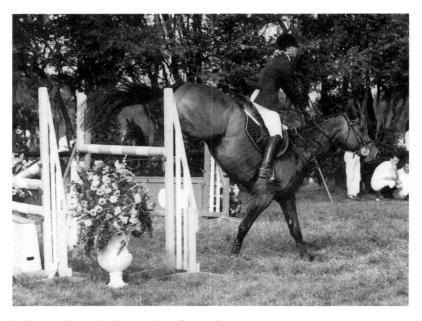

Fig. 12.34 Landing with rider: non-lead foreleg impact

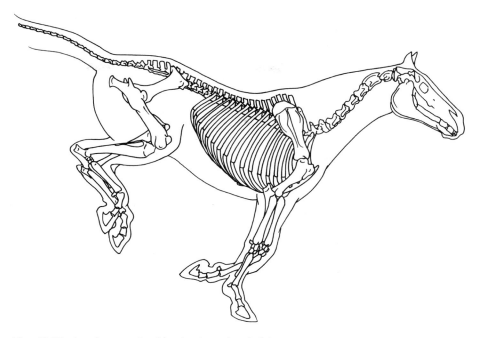

Fig. 12.35   Landing: non-lead foreleg impact – skeleton

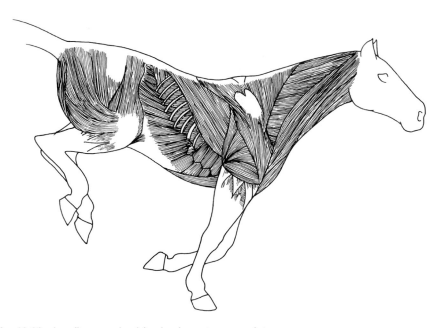

Fig. 12.36   Landing: non-lead foreleg impact – musculature

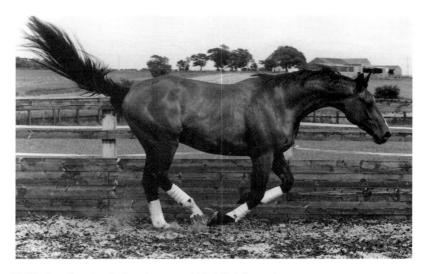

Fig. 12.37   Landing: forelimb getaway and hind limb impact

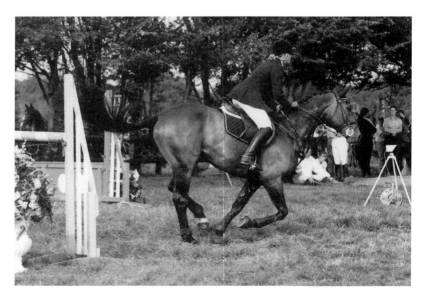

Fig. 12.38   Landing with rider: forelimb getaway and hind limb impact

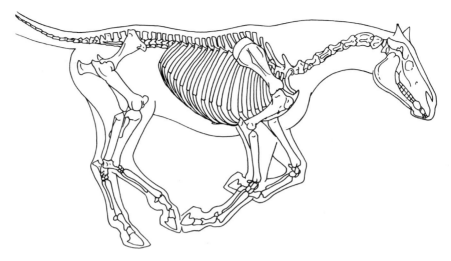

Fig. 12.39   Landing: forelimb getaway and hind limb impact – skeleton

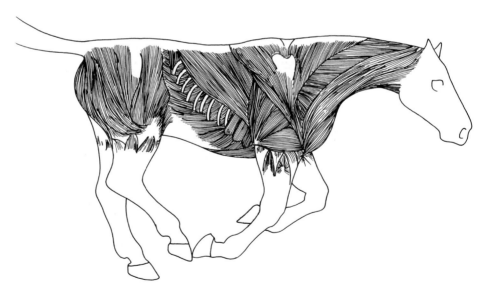

Fig. 12.40   Landing: forelimb getaway and hind limb impact – musculature

The getaway (Figs 12.41–12.43)

The two hind feet power the horse forward and the front feet bound ahead with the non-lead (left) fore making first contact with the ground. Providing the horse has landed in a balanced manner the canter is now resumed.

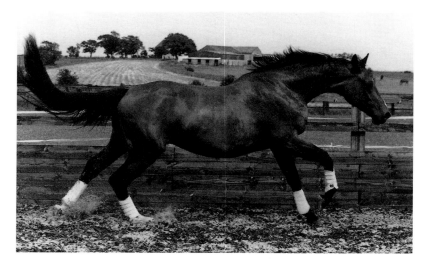

Fig. 12.41 The getaway

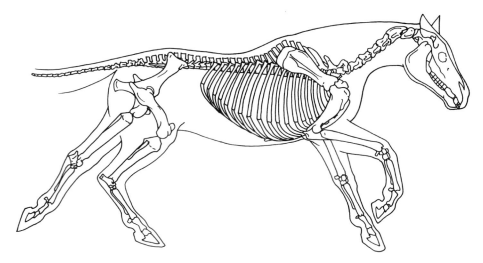

Fig. 12.42 The getaway – skeleton

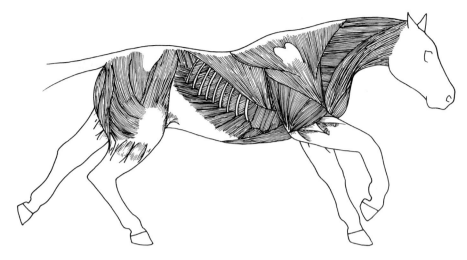

Fig. 12.43   The getaway – musculature

The ideal jumper

Although successful equine athletes come in all shapes and sizes, from a biomechanical point of view the ideal conformation for jumping is as follows:

- Long, slim limbs
- A light, streamlined body
- Powerful hindquarters
- A light forehand
- A well laid back shoulder
- Sound legs and feet.

It is difficult for horses with a large head and forehand to form the ideal shape over a fence – they tend to take off and descend steeply and land heavily.

Evaluating jumping technique

However good the horse's conformation, it is essential that the horse has a good jumping technique and is careful. To cope with big fences jumping has to be easy for the horse. Many event horses do not have as good a technique as showjumpers – it is more important for them to be bold and fast – and they may find the showjumping phase of the competition particularly difficult. It is useful to evaluate the horse's jumping technique both loose and with a rider. The following points should be observed:

- Over the jump the head should be lowered, the withers raised and the back rounded
- The forelimbs should be tightly folded as a pair. The horse should not dangle a knee or foot
- The knee and forearm should be brought up higher than the point of shoulder
- The hind limbs should also be folded as a pair
- The joints of the hind limb should be able to open up so that the hindquarters can be flicked up and over the fence
- The horse should learn from its mistakes
- The horse should be confident at jumping
- The horse should be able to adjust his stride to find a consistently secure take-off zone.

Chapter 13

Rolling and shaking

Rolling behaviour

In the horse rolling is a form of grooming. One of the objects of rolling is to provide a protective layer of mud or dust. In the winter a thick layer of mud serves to insulate the horse from the cold and to protect its skin from the rain. Rain-sodden skin is prone to mud fever and rain scald. In the summer, a layer of dust on the coat helps to give some protection from the irritating bites of flies and midges and discourages skin parasites. Horses will sometimes paw the ground before rolling and this may be to disturb dust and mud for them to roll in.

Figure 13.1 shows the rolling sequence. The horse lies down in the normal fashion and then kicks itself over onto its back and rubs its back against the ground whilst keeping its feet in the air. After several rubs it rolls back onto its side again, either the same side or the other side from which it started. The horse then rises, stands with all four limbs slightly splayed, and shakes its body vigorously from head to hind limbs. This shaking is an action pattern referred to as the 'wet dog shake' and makes the skin ripple all over the body, removing the dirt and debris picked up while the horse was rolling. Behaviourists regard rolling and shaking as a 'compound action pattern' and, as such, it can only be fully performed in the field or other outdoor area. It is essential for the psychological well-being of a horse that it is allowed periodic freedom to indulge in this important natural behaviour.

The back and rump are areas that the horse cannot reach except by grooming from another horse or by rolling. The stabled or rugged horse cannot be groomed by a companion so it is little wonder that often the first thing a stabled horse does when it is turned out is to roll. Horses clearly enjoy rolling and they often roll after exercise when they are hot and itchy. However, the grass-kept horse will also roll just for fun.

Colic

Horses often roll if they are experiencing abdominal discomfort, and excessive rolling is a typical sign that a horse is suffering from colic. Characteristically, the horse looks round at its side, paws the ground and gets up and down frequently. Where the pain is severe the horse will roll

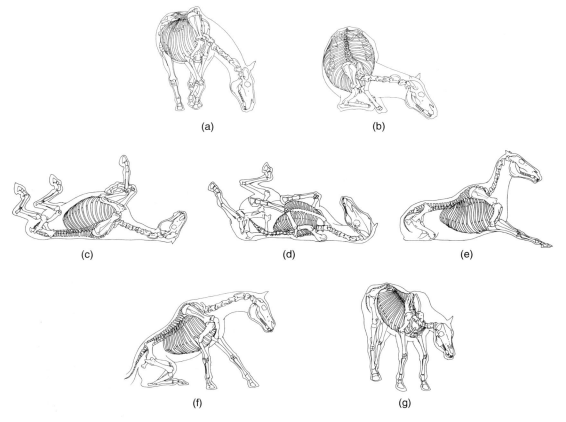

Fig. 13.1   Rolling sequence

violently, thrashing its head and legs against the ground. When watching
the horse's limbs and head flailing against the ground while the horse is
rolling, it is easy to visualise the damage that the horse with colic can
inflict on itself.

Preferred rolling places
Horses usually choose one or two preferred rolling spots and this may
help to establish herd bonding by coating them in the 'herd smell'. Wild
horses and zebras have rolling rituals, with herd members taking turns
to use the rolling spot.

Scenting
Stabled horses often paw the bed and roll when they are put into a new
stable or if clean bedding has been put down. It is thought that they do
this to cover the bedding with their own smell.

The rolling sequence

Getting down (Figs 13.2–13.7)

The horse begins the rolling sequence by starting to lie down as it normally would. The horse lowers its head right down to the ground, moving the centre of gravity both forwards and down. The hind legs are moved forwards underneath the body and the horse begins to bend at the knees (Figs 13.2–13.4).

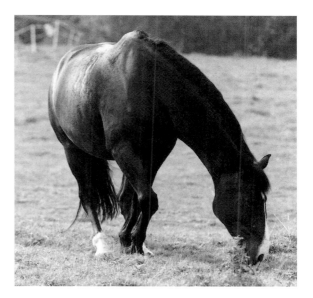

Fig. 13.2   Bending the knees

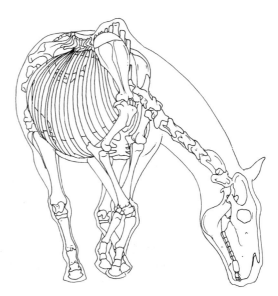

Fig. 13.3   Bending the knees – skeleton

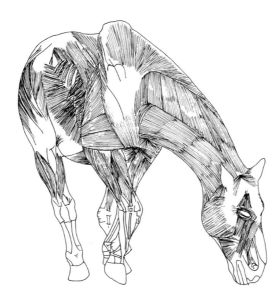

Fig. 13.4 Bending the knees – musculature

The stance is highly characteristic, and if a ridden horse begins to get down, the rider can feel the horse's posture change and must ride the horse forwards quickly. Frequently, hot sweaty ponies find the temptation to roll almost irresistible and must be watched carefully all the time they are halted if their young riders are to avoid embarrassment!

The horse gently lowers itself to its knees, folding the lower leg underneath its chest (Figs 13.5–13.7). At the same time the hocks and stifles flex, allowing the hindquarters to sink. Once the horse has achieved this position it lets its body and hindquarters flop onto the ground.

The ribs and pelvis

The unusual angle in Fig. 13.6 shows the both the spring of the ribs and the position of the pelvis, which can be seen behind the ribcage. In the standing horse it is hard to appreciate the size of these structures, and it is only when the horse is rolling or lying down that the size becomes apparent.

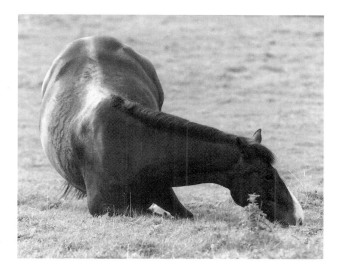

Fig. 13.5   Front end down

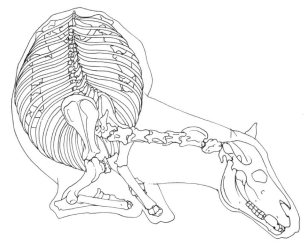

Fig. 13.6   Front end down – skeleton

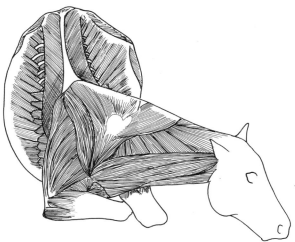

Fig. 13.7   Front end down – musculature

Rolling over (Figs 13.8–13.13)

Once the horse is down it lets itself fall to one side. It then rubs the side of its head, neck and body before kicking powerfully against the ground to roll over onto its back. Once on its back the horse rubs its back and rump against the ground (Fig. 13.8).

Many horses will have a preferred side on which they get down first. Some horses are able to roll over to the other side (Fig. 13.11), whereas others have to get up, then get down again to groom the other side. These horses sometimes only roll on one side or the other. Those that find rolling over easy may roll back and forth several times before they get up. It is said to be the sign of an athletic horse with good conformation that is free from back pain, if it can roll right over. However, overweight horses and those with very high withers may not be able to do this.

The pelvis

It is difficult to visualise the anatomy of the pelvis from two-dimensional diagrams and from looking at the horse from the side. At the top of the hindquarters is the croup (tuber sacrale), below that is the point of the hip (tuber coxae) and below that the hip joint where the femur articulates with the pelvis. From the angle shown in Fig. 13.12 it is easier to see the pelvis as a ring of bone, attaching to the spine and hind limbs. Fig. 13.12 also shows a clear view of the horse's sternum. From Fig. 13.13 it is possible to appreciate the sheer size of the muscles of the upper thigh and area occupied by the gut, where there is little skeletal muscle.

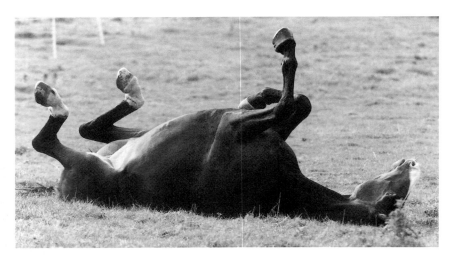

Fig. 13.8   Equine bliss! The horse rolls onto its back.

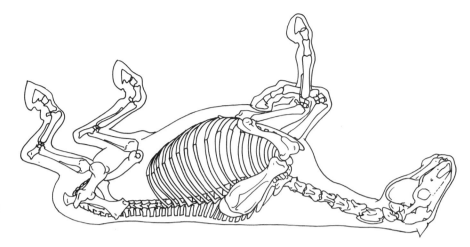

Fig. 13.9 Rolling on to its back – skeleton

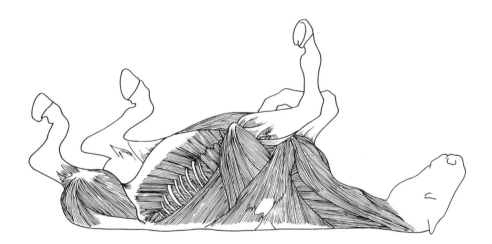

Fig. 13.10 Rolling on to its back – musculature

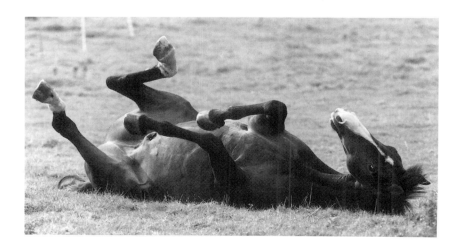

Fig. 13.11 Rolling back over

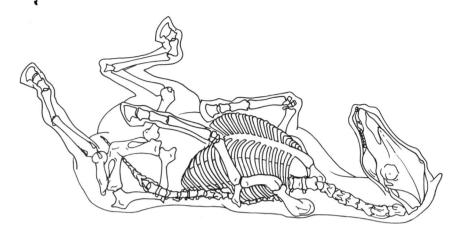

Fig. 13.12   Rolling back over – skeleton

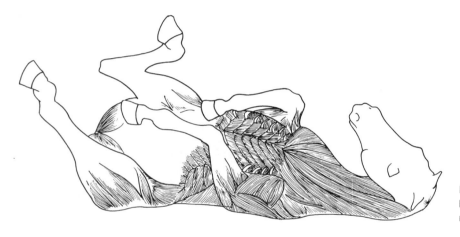

Fig. 13.13   Rolling back over – musculature

Getting the front end up (Figs 13.14–13.19)

To rise, the horse manoeuvres both front legs out from under its body and places them in front. Sometimes the horse will rest in this position and even stretch the front legs and head and neck (Fig. 13.14). To get the front end off the ground and move the hind legs underneath the body, the horse raises its head and neck and slides its front legs out in front of its chest and forces them against the ground (Figs 13.14, 13.17). A slippery surface therefore makes it hard for the horse to get up.

With a lurch the horse levers its forehand off the ground before it is able to raise its hindquarters. A great deal of effort is required, but some horses are more nimble and find getting up easier than others. As a creature of flight, not fight, the horse instinctively feels vulnerable when it is lying down. This is compounded by the effort the horse has to make when it gets up. The stabled horse will only lie down when it feels safe and secure.

Cattle lie down and get up in a different way from horses. They lie down haunches first and get up haunches first.

Sitting on the head

To get up, the horse has to lift its head and neck. Therefore, if a horse has to be kept recumbent for any reason, it is possible to keep it down by 'sitting on its head'. The handler should stand behind the horse's head and then kneel on the horse's poll. If the horse is very strong and the handler light, the handler can also bend forwards and use their hands to keep the horse's nose on the floor. In this position the handler can quickly get out of the horse's way and not be struck by the front feet when the horse is allowed to rise.

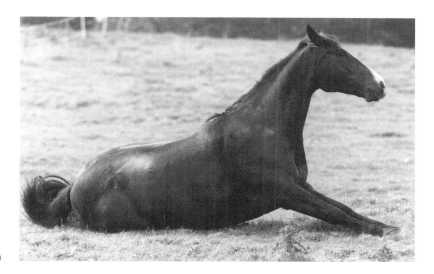

Fig. 13.14 A quick stretch

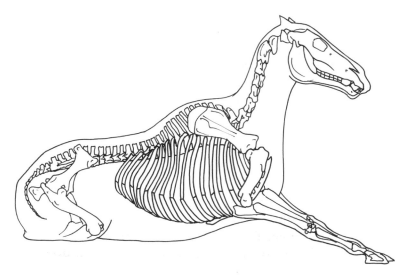

Fig. 13.15 A quick stretch – skeleton

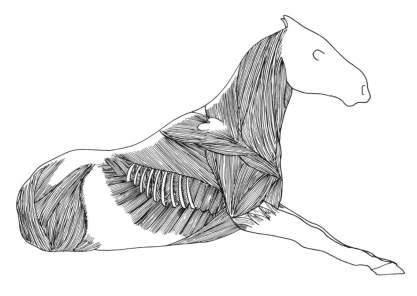

Fig. 13.16   A quick stretch
– musculature

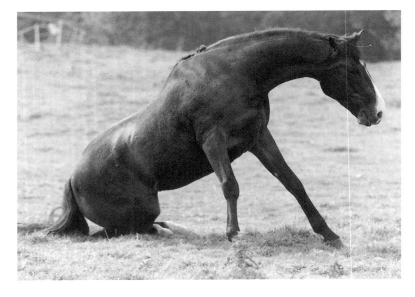

Fig. 13.17   Getting the front
end up

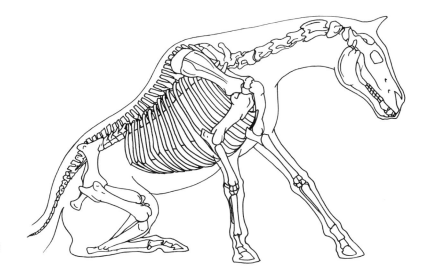

Fig. 13.18   Getting the front
end up – skeleton

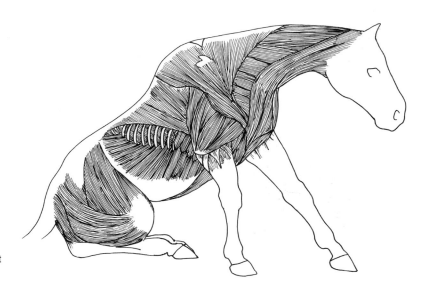

Fig. 13.19   Getting the front
end up – musculature

Shaking

Rolling and shaking are associated behaviours. The healthy horse should shake after getting up. Failure to do so may mean that the horse is rolling due to pain rather than pleasure.

The mechanics of shaking (Figs 13.20–13.22)

Horses can shake very vigorously. In Fig. 13.20 the horse has relaxed the stay apparatus of the forelimb and has started the shaking process with the head and neck. The energetic shaking of the neck passes to the relaxed forelimbs, causing them to buckle and wobble. Figure 13.20 shows how little weight is being taken on the front legs. The forelimbs straighten as the shake passes along the trunk to the hindquarters. Figure 13.20 also gives an unusual view of the horse's neck muscles flopping from side to side, and the position of the cervical vertebrae in Fig. 13.21 clearly shows why this happens.

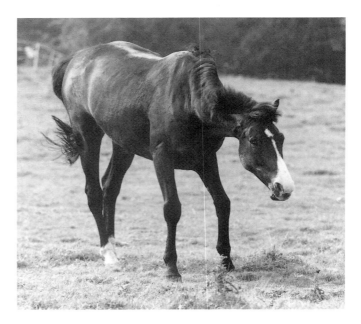

Fig. 13.20   A good shake!

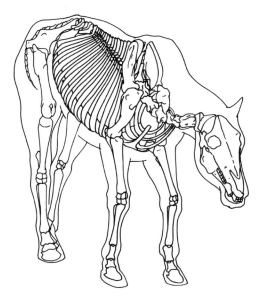

Fig. 13.21 Shaking – skeleton

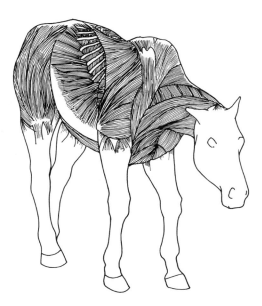

Fig. 13.22 Shaking – musculature

Index